THE HEALTH
OF PEOPLE

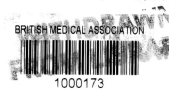

The Campaign for Social Science was launched in 2011 by the Academy of Social Sciences to promote social science to the UK Government and the wider public. We campaign for policies that support social science inquiry in the UK, such as the retention of large-scale longitudinal research programmes.

The Health of People is the successor report to *The Business of People: The Significance of Social Science Over The Next Decade*, published in 2015 as the basis of our advocacy on behalf of the social sciences and making recommendations – on research funding, social science capacity and use of expert advice by government – to maximise social science's contribution.

THE HEALTH OF PEOPLE

HOW THE SOCIAL SCIENCES CAN IMPROVE POPULATION HEALTH

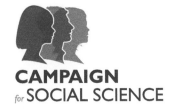

CAMPAIGN
for SOCIAL SCIENCE

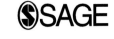

Los Angeles | London | New Delhi
Singapore | Washington DC | Melbourne

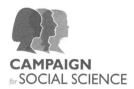

CAMPAIGN
for SOCIAL SCIENCE

33 Finsbury Square
London
EC2A 1AG

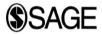

Los Angeles | London | New Delhi
Singapore | Washington DC | Melbourne

SAGE Publications Ltd
1 Oliver's Yard
55 City Road
London EC1Y 1SP

SAGE Publications Inc.
2455 Teller Road
Thousand Oaks, California 91320

SAGE Publications India Pvt Ltd
B 1/I 1 Mohan Cooperative Industrial Area
Mathura Road
New Delhi 110 044

SAGE Publications Asia-Pacific Pte Ltd
3 Church Street
#10-04 Samsung Hub
Singapore 049483

Editor: Judi Burger
Production editor: Victoria Nicholas
Marketing manager: Susheel Gokarakonda
Cover design: Wendy Scott
Typeset by: C&M Digitals (P) Ltd, Chennai,
India
Printed by CPI Group (UK) Ltd, Croydon, CR0 4YY

British Library Cataloguing in Publication data

A catalogue record for this book is available from
the British Library

ISBN 978-1-47398-945-0 (pbk)

At SAGE we take sustainability seriously. Most of our products are printed in the UK using FSC papers and boards.
When we print overseas we ensure sustainable papers are used as measured by the PREPS grading system.
We undertake an annual audit to monitor our sustainability.

CONTENTS

Forewords   vii
Acknowledgements   ix
Scope of this report   xi
Executive summary   xiii
Recommendations   xv

Introduction   1
Healthy behaviour: Promoting population behaviour change   7
Understanding behaviour change   15
Strategies to encourage and support changes in
health-related behaviours   19
Self-management of illness and long-term conditions   23
Behaviour change and implications for health
service delivery   29
Social science and new ways of configuring services   35
Social science and data   41
Recommendations   49

Appendix A: Contributors   61
References   65

FOREWORDS

This report is very welcome and timely. The contributions of modern science and technology to the quality of modern healthcare are everywhere visible. They include non-invasive imaging, minimalist surgery and new anaesthetics, stents and statins, genetic testing and new techniques and treatments for cancers. There is much more to come as we head into the era of personalised medicine in which diagnostics and treatments are moulded with much greater accuracy around the individual.

Less obvious, but equally as important, has been the contribution of the social sciences, as evidenced by the examples in this report. Healthcare is enormously expensive. Relatively few nations have even a basic model of universal healthcare coverage that provides equity of access to an entire population, let alone with the NHS promise of being free at the point of clinical need. And no such nation has a model that is economically sustainable well into the future, given demographic changes and rising costs, as science enables us to perform life-saving procedures that were previously impossible, and as public expectations rise accordingly. Across all of these domains lie the social sciences.

More importantly for healthcare systems across the world is the improvement of population health, primarily through the prevention of ill-health, but also through shifting presentation, diagnosis and treatment further upstream, so that healthy lives are prolonged and healthcare becomes more than simply a patch and repair service for acute and chronic conditions.

This report proposes a number of steps towards a more coherent and focused approach in linking the social and behavioural sciences to these ends, and is to be warmly welcomed and applauded. It's a strong case and there is an urgent need.

Sir Malcolm Grant CBE FAcSS
Chair, NHS England

The Campaign for Social Science was set up in 2011 to inform public policy, build coalitions and engage in measured advocacy. It sprang from the Academy of Social Sciences, which now has a fellowship of around 1,100 eminent academics and practitioners across universities, business, government and civil society. 42 learned societies are also members, representing over 90,000 social scientists in all walks of life.

In 2015, ahead of the last general election, we published *The Business of People*, to highlight the contributions of the social sciences to the myriad economic, social and environmental challenges which confront the UK and the wider world.

This successor report – *The Health of People* – represents a timely intervention in policy and public debates about the health and wellbeing of our society. From transforming health services to influencing health-related behaviours, the report makes clear that too much of the potential of social science still lies untapped. And it makes a set of clear recommendations to improve the provision, transmission and uptake of research evidence in ways that can make tangible improvements to population health.

I would like to extend my warmest thanks to those who have devoted time to the project over the past year, especially to Professor Susan Michie FAcSS, who expended considerable time and energy in expertly steering the report through to completion, and the members of her Working Group, as well as to our Review Group, whose experience and insights provided a valuable reality check on our conclusions. Let me also thank Sharon Witherspoon MBE FAcSS and Daniela Puska of the Campaign team, and Professor Jon Glasby FAcSS, a member of our Board, all of whom made important contributions to the drafting of the report and management of the project.

Finally, we are grateful to Ziyad Marar and colleagues at SAGE Publishing for their ongoing partnership and for publishing the report; and to the Association of the British Pharmaceutical Industry (ABPI), British Psychological Society, Cancer Research UK, Nesta, Society for the Study of Addiction, and Wellcome Trust for their generous support.

We are in a period of transition, both within the NHS and wider health system, and across UK universities and research. Reports like this, and the wider efforts of the Campaign to demonstrate how social science can help to meet our shared priorities, have never been more urgently required.

James Wilsdon

Professor James Wilsdon FAcSS
Chair, Campaign for Social Science
campaign.chair@acss.org.uk

ACKNOWLEDGEMENTS

WORKING GROUP

Susan Michie FAcSS (Chair), Professor of Health Psychology and Director of the Centre for Behaviour Change, University College London; **Gwyn Bevan**, Professor of Policy Analysis and Director of the MSc in Public Management and Governance, London School of Economics and Political Science; **Rona Campbell** FAcSS, Professor of Public Health Research, University of Bristol; **Joanna Coast**, Professor in the Economics of Health & Care, University of Bristol; **Simon Christmas**, Visiting Senior Research Fellow, King's College London; **Robbie Foy**, Professor of Primary Care, Leeds Institute of Health Sciences, and a General Practitioner; **Jon Glasby** FAcSS, Head of the School of Social Policy, University of Birmingham; **Ann Hoskins**, Independent Public Health Consultant; **Marie Johnston** FAcSS, Professor of Health Psychology, University of Aberdeen; **Mike Kelly**, Professor and Senior Visiting Fellow in the Department of Public Health and Primary Care, University of Cambridge; **Lawrence King**, Professor of Political Economy and Sociology, University of Cambridge; **Theresa Marteau** FAcSS, Professor and Director of the Behaviour and Health Research Unit, University of Cambridge; **Matt Sutton**, Professor of Health Economics, University of Manchester; **Robert West**, Professor of Health Psychology and Director of Tobacco Studies, University College London; **Tim Whitaker** FAcSS, Director of Communications, Hanover Housing Association; **Sally Wyke**, Deputy Director and Interdisciplinary Research Professor at the Institute of Health and Wellbeing, University of Glasgow; **Dagmar Zeuner**, Director of Public Health, London Borough of Merton.

REVIEW PANEL

Ian Dodge, National Director for Commissioning Strategy, NHS England; **Carol Tannahill** FAcSS, Director, Glasgow Centre for Population Health and Chief Social Policy Adviser; **Sir John Tooke**, Executive Chairman and Founder, Academic Health Solutions.

WITH THANKS TO

Particular thanks to Sharon Witherspoon MBE FAcSS, and also to Stephen Anderson, Daniela Puska, Alessandro Lanuto, Helen Spriggs and Sam Martin at the Campaign for Social Science, David Walker FAcSS and Roses Leech-Wilkinson, as well as Nicola Gale, Russell Mannion, Rachel Posaner, Christian Bohm and David Evans for comments and support with an early draft of this report.

The many people who contributed to the report through roundtable discussions and the Call for Evidence are acknowledged at the back of the report.

The report is kindly supported by the British Psychological Society, Cancer Research UK, Nesta, SAGE Publishing, Society for the Study of Addiction, The Association of the British Pharmaceutical Industry, and the Wellcome Trust.

SCOPE OF THIS REPORT

This report is concerned with how the social sciences can help improve population health. While biomedical sciences are primary drivers of health treatments and health-care, the social sciences have an important role in informing and helping change the environments, policies, practices and behaviours that influence the health of people.

We use the term 'health' to cover wellbeing and mental health, as well as physical health. We also acknowledge that health and social care are interdependent: the one needs to be considered in the light of the other. We use the term 'social sciences' to cover a wide range of academic disciplines, including psychology, anthropology, political science, sociology, economics and geography. We sometimes talk about the 'social sciences' and sometimes 'the social and behavioural sciences'. When we use the longer phrase, it is to remind readers that social sciences include distinctive approaches to human behaviour, emphasising that if we are to improve population health, we need a comprehensive approach to behaviour change, drawing on the full gamut of theories, evidence and methodologies from the social and behavioural sciences.

The term 'behavioral' refers to overt actions; to underlying psychological processes such as cognition, emotion, temperament, and motivation; and to bio-behavioral interactions. The term 'social' encompasses sociocultural, socioeconomic, and socio-demographic status; to biosocial interactions; and to the various levels of social context from small groups to complex cultural systems and societal influences. The core areas of behavioral and social sciences research are those that have a major and explicit focus on the understanding of behavioral or social processes, or on the use of these processes to predict or influence health outcomes or health risk factors.[1]

This report has as one of its major themes the importance of the social sciences in achieving behaviour change; it also acknowledges the importance of social sciences in improving health in other ways: by describing the social and economic determinants of health inequalities, helping understand economic factors in health and healthcare, and so on. But this is not an attempt at an exhaustive account of how the social sciences have contributed to improvements in health. Instead it is a short report on how the current relationship between the social sciences, health policies and interventions and health could be improved for the health of people.

This report is timely in that it is published soon after a report from the Academy of Medical Sciences, *Improving the Health of the Public by 2040*. Our recommendations complement theirs and, together, the recommendations form a solid basis for action that could transform the health of people in the UK.[2]

EXECUTIVE SUMMARY

This report examines the current and potential role of social and behavioural sciences in improving population health, with health considered in its broadest sense to include wellbeing and mental health. It argues that while the social sciences are already making a contribution, this needs to go further if we are to tackle the challenges of improving population health. This use should include population-level changes in policy and practice to improve health, by environmental changes as well as promoting health-related behaviours, such as self-management of long-term conditions, and the practices of health providers and planners. Effective interventions are those that recognise the systems within which health and ill-health occur and those that need to change to achieve improvements. Change is needed at many levels: for example, in the behaviours of health service planners and those delivering services. We present case studies to show what has been achieved but also point to how much more could be done if social sciences were more systematically involved in health policy and practice.

Attempts to change behaviour are often based upon 'common sense,' flawed assumptions about how people behave and unrealistically optimistic interpretations of limited evidence. For example, strategies relying on provision of information or guidelines alone seldom result in significant change but are often used despite repeated failures of this approach.

This report argues that the social sciences provide models and methods for a more comprehensive and coherent approach to behaviour and behaviour change that takes account of the physical and social context, physical and psychological capability, and people's 'reflective' and 'automatic' motivational processes. Long-term maintenance of change is key to improving health and the factors that influence this often differ from those that trigger short-term change. The social sciences provide a wide range of methods for developing and evaluating interventions and frameworks that can be tailored to health needs and practical circumstances. The report makes the case that the development of a national strategy for accelerating advances in the social and behavioural sciences, and for embedding the translation of these advances into policy and practice, would be a sound investment in the health of people.

RECOMMENDATIONS

1. RECOMMENDATIONS FOR COORDINATING AND FUNDING RESEARCH AND IMPLEMENTATION

1.1 We call for a UK strategic coordinating body for research into population health. It should bring together major research funders (such as National Institute for Health Research (NIHR), Medical Research Council (MRC), the Economic and Social Research Council (ESRC), Wellcome Trust, Cancer Research UK, and British Heart Foundation), public health bodies (such as Public Health England, Health Protection Scotland, Public Health Wales, Public Health Agency for Northern Ireland, NHS England, Scotland, Wales and Northern Ireland), and relevant learned societies (such as the Academy of Social Sciences and Academy of Medical Sciences).[3]

1.2 This coordinating body should take as its remit a wide view of population health and approaches to improving it, recognising (i) the role of behaviour in improving health and the environmental and social systems within which behaviour occurs and changes, and (ii) the diversity of change agents at population, community and individual level influencing health indirectly as well as directly. Its aim should be to support high-quality, multi-disciplinary research on these issues and on how best to translate research evidence into policy and practice.

1.3 One of the new body's first tasks should be to commission a review of the existing infrastructure for health research, including social and behavioural research and its implementation in healthcare and public health,

involving stakeholders, funders, and major research centres. This review should examine research funding, funding agencies, funding mechanisms, and infrastructure for implementation at national, regional and local level, including resources and roles dedicated to this.

1.4 **The review should make recommendations regarding the building of an integrated system for multi-disciplinary research and implementation.** This would include reviewing existing centres and networks, addressing the weaknesses in the current approaches while building on their strengths, to ensure critical mass and stability.

1.5 **The review should consider establishing a number of 'implementation laboratories'.** These would focus on the development and evaluation of implementation strategies for the health service, local government and other parts of society relevant to health.

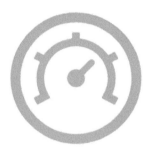

2. RECOMMENDATIONS FOR CAPACITY BUILDING

2.1 **The UK strategic coordinating body should review the existing skills and expertise available for research into behavioural and social sciences in relation to health.** This review should assess how the necessary skills and expertise can be developed, including the need for more diverse and appropriate training pathways, and include training in how to engage effectively with potential users of research, as well as how medical researchers and practitioners (including Directors of Public Health, service commissioners, and managers) could engage more strategically with social science expertise.

2.2 **The UK strategic coordinating body should consider how best to encourage and incentivise those involved in promoting health and commissioning and delivering healthcare services** to make appropriate use of research findings and expertise, including social science evidence. In doing so, it should make use of behavioural and social science research about incentivisation and research translation.

2.3 **We recommend that the strategy for capacity building should include developing greater numbers of people who can ally high-level data and informatics skills with substantive knowledge of health research.**[4] This will require a strategic priority among research funders and a focus on training pathways to provide new capacity, and include consideration of how to draw mathematics, physics and data analytic specialists into social and behavioural health and health delivery research.

2.4 We recommend that all research funders consider a new interdisciplinary research agenda on the importance of macro- and micro-environments and of social relationships (including the roles of changing social norms and social support) in bringing about behaviour change.

3. RECOMMENDATIONS FOR DATA PROVISION AND ACCESS

3.1 We support the calls of the Wachter review[5] for the development of efficient and effective systems for collecting data relevant to behaviour change in healthcare and public health. The use of such data (usually in the form of de-personalised data sets, where individuals are not identifiable) is essential for public-benefit research to improve the health of the nation.

3.2 The UK strategic coordinating body should play an active role in unlocking the current difficulties in accessing health data and linking them to social data to provide research access that is both necessary to improve population health and consistent with public acceptance of public-benefit research carried out with appropriate safeguards.

3.3 We also call for a greater urgency in the deliberations of NHS Digital and the Department of Health over health data linkage and for the 'social consent' model we propose in this report to form an important foundation for these policy discussions.

3.4 We recommend that parliamentarians, policy-makers, health organisations and the broader public should be engaged in an urgent debate about the benefits of opening up access to link 'de-personalised' health data with broader social data to improve health policy, practice and behaviour. Social scientists should be active participants in these discussions about data linkage, as they have useful research and evidence about public views on these matters.

INTRODUCTION

The discoveries that tobacco smoking causes lung cancer, a retrovirus causes AIDS, or that cervical cancer is caused by a papillomavirus, do not by themselves improve human health. Human behaviours such as smoking, drug use, sexual activity and relationships, or uptake of screening do not change instantly in response to such discoveries.

Rather such behaviours are embedded in social relationships, and are subject to norms, values and social meanings, and the way we organise our society. If we are to improve population health and reduce inequalities in health, we need to understand these behaviours better, and how to change them.

We also need to understand that these behaviours are not a matter of simple or rational choices ('surely if we tell people to stop smoking, or to take more exercise, or have fewer babies, they will?'), and that research on social aspects of health and illness is therefore as important as studying the biological processes.

Professor Dame Sally Macintyre DBE[6]

The health of people often calls to mind the delivery of healthcare – by GPs, hospital specialists and health professionals in social care and community settings, especially for older or disabled people. The social sciences of all forms have made important contributions to improving healthcare delivery, and we draw attention to some of these in this report.

But many important improvements in population health result from changes in people's behaviour, whether they are patients, health professionals or members of the public. These rarely arise simply from education or by the provision of information, important though these are. Instead they arise from a multiplicity of factors relating to motivation, capability and the physical or social environment – for example, changes in law, changes in what is considered acceptable, and environmental changes that make behaviour change easier. The social sciences have played their part in helping to document this and to understand how interventions achieve their effects and therefore to improve the design of interventions and policies. A good example of this is England's Comprehensive Tobacco Control Strategy, which included interventions and policies at many levels, including introducing legislation for smoke-free public places, changing taxation and packaging, and providing evidence-based services for those trying to quit.[7] The evidence for many of these policies arose from the social and behavioural sciences.

So the health of people in the United Kingdom already depends on social science methods and evidence. Whether it takes the form of planning for an ageing population in delivering health services, examining the economic costs of different medical treatments, delivering preventative actions to support healthy ageing, examining how diseases and behaviours are spread through the population, or understanding how to change behaviours of health professionals and healthcare practices, the social sciences are essential to modern healthcare delivery and to population health more generally. Understanding the economic costs and benefits of clinical and population health interventions, both in the short term and the long term, underpins modern health and social care planning. Better understanding of clinical outcomes – of treatment patterns, hospital procedures and even of different hospitals' and doctors' practices – helps drive improvements in patient health. And better understanding of how the behaviour of people – patients, health professionals, commissioners, citizens and communities – can change their practices to produce better health outcomes is now receiving growing attention.

According to many international comparisons, the UK National Health Services are among the best in the developed world in terms of quality of care, access and efficiency. Of 11 high-income countries reviewed by the Commonwealth Fund in 2014, the UK came top in terms of effective care, safe care, coordinated care and patient-centred care, second (behind Sweden) in terms of equity, and third in terms of timeliness of care.[8] This was, of course, before the pressures of the last few years, when UK healthcare spending has dropped as a proportion of GDP and the growth in health spending has been lower than its post-war average and lower than the growth in age-related needs.[9]

By contrast, in the same study by The Commonwealth Fund, the UK came second from last in terms of 'healthy lives', where the UK was ranked behind all the other countries surveyed apart from the United States. This last category was measured according to three indicators (mortality amenable to healthcare; infant mortality; and healthy life expectancy), with the authors acknowledging that these factors are influenced more by broader social and economic factors than by treatment services. Other countries may have healthier populations or less socio-economic inequality that leads to ill-health.[10]

Indeed, one of the signal contributions of much recent social science research has been to demonstrate how much people's health is related to social and economic factors (for example, housing, employment, the built environment and nutrition), as demonstrated by research led by Professor Sir Michael Marmot,[11] and illustrated in Figure 1.

The need for action to address these social factors has been acknowledged by the National Institute for Health and Care Excellence (NICE).[12] They are important both as causes of ill-health, and as drivers of collective and individual behaviours. Health-related behaviours have become an increasingly important focus of policy in the context of the challenges arising from an ageing population,[13] the growing rates of population obesity,[14] and an increasing number of people with chronic conditions such as diabetes that require long-term treatment and management.[15] It is clear that acute healthcare services cannot tackle these alone.

Figure I   The multi-level influences on human behaviour and health

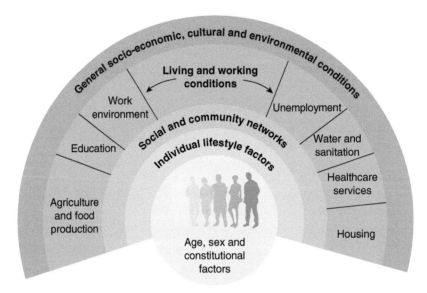

Source: Dahigren and Whitehead, 1991

These pressures are acknowledged by the NHS England *Five Year Forward View* where it stated:

> The NHS has dramatically improved over the past fifteen years. Cancer and cardiac out-comes are better; waits are shorter; patient satisfaction much higher. Progress has con-tinued even during global recession and austerity thanks to protected funding and the commitment of NHS staff. But quality of care can be variable, preventable illness is wide-spread, health inequalities deep-rooted. Our patients' needs are changing, new treatment options are emerging, and we face particular challenges in areas such as mental health, cancer and support for frail older patients. Service pressures are building. ... If the nation fails to get serious about prevention then recent progress in healthy life expectancies will stall, health inequalities will widen, and our ability to fund beneficial new treatments will be crowded-out by the need to spend billions of pounds on wholly avoidable illness.[16]

Challenges of health-related behaviours face health and social care systems across countries with developed economies and modern healthcare, though often to different degrees. These include behavioural factors (such as physical inactivity, smoking, alcohol consumption), social inequalities which generate these and other risks to healthcare, rising obesity levels, and the challenges of delivering health and social care to an ageing population.[17] Other challenges are 'income effects' (the fact that demand for spending on health tends to rise as incomes rise) and the costs of adopting technological and medical advances, which, as the Office for Budget Responsibility has recently argued, are as important as demography in driving up healthcare costs.[18]

In the light of this, a current priority of policy-makers is to understand and promote changes in health-related behaviours – by patients, the public and healthcare providers. The social sciences can contribute to avoiding errors that policy-makers and politicians frequently make in efforts to bring about behaviour change.[19] They can do this by *description* – asking what is going on; by *explanation* – understanding what interventions may work or what causes change in this setting; and by helping inform *implementation* of evidence into policy and practice and *generalisation* across contexts.

There is growing awareness in a number of quarters that addressing health challenges will require greater attention to interventions that can alter behaviour both to address healthcare delivery and improve population health through prevention.[20] In the UK, recent initiatives include a programme of work led by Public Health England;[21] those led by Nesta, which has now set up a Health Lab with a focus largely on behavioural change;[22] and projects led by the Behavioural Insights Team.[23]

The issues addressed in this report are similar to many of those examined by the Academy of Medical Sciences (AMS) in its report *Improving the Health of the Public by 2040: Optimising the research environment for a healthier, fairer future.*[24] That report argued for more and better multi-disciplinary research, including the social and behavioural sciences, to improve population health and healthcare. The current report echoes and expands on many of its recommendations. In particular, we welcome the recommendations that the UK needs more social and behavioural research on disease prevention as a means of improving health, and on evaluation of how to change health service delivery; that the UK needs more strategic coordination and more funding of public health and health improvement research; and that the UK would benefit from better use of data to improve population health. The AMS report also calls for trans-disciplinary approaches to improving population health, that is, going beyond disciplines working alongside each other to creating new knowledge as a result of disciplines sharing and learning from each other's methods, theories and knowledge. Here, we outline some particular contributions of the social sciences.

This report sets out a vision of the ways in which better use of the social and behavioural sciences can help improve the health of people, in part by improving the prospects of developing a more complete strategy for promoting health and wellbeing to avoid the need for healthcare. It examines the use of social science methods and findings in: (i) changing and maintaining health-related behaviours by individuals, and in communities and populations; (ii) healthcare planning and health service delivery; and

(iii) the use of data. In each of these areas, it gives examples of how these sciences have already made a contribution.

The aim of the report is not merely to describe some of the contributions currently being made by the social sciences; it is also to argue that we need a substantial increase in the role of social sciences if we are to address many of the challenges of modern healthcare.

This report provides arguments, alongside evidence, that we need to build capacity – both in human skills and expertise, and in our institutions – and a more complete incorporation of robust social science evidence and methods into developing health and social policies and in the delivery of health and social interventions. We put forward recommendations that, if enacted, would strengthen the use and impact of social and behavioural sciences in improving individual, community and population health and in translating research evidence into healthcare delivery and other pathways to health. They also take account of what we know about how to achieve change – both in how individuals behave and in how organisations and communities function. There is wide debate about the value and efficacy of health-based interventions that target individual behaviour and those that focus on community and cultural values. For example, there is a strong case for community-led participatory health research producing more enduring results, especially where communities are empowered to take control of factors that affect health outcomes, and so reduce inequalities in health.[25]

Many of these ideas have been discussed in round-table meetings with health policy-makers, practitioners and researchers (see Appendix A). They involve practical suggestions about how the social sciences can play their part in improving the health of people.

We also make the case that there is a pressing need to develop skills and infrastructures to promote the engagement of all healthcare professions, healthcare and social services and population health strategies with a robust culture of social science innovation, experiment and broader evaluation, and for social scientists to improve and deepen their own skills and expertise.

An important issue that is beyond the scope of this report is how the economic and political situation in the UK influences health and healthcare. These considerations provide the context for the current report but the report itself is concerned with how the health of people can be maximised by effective use of the social sciences within the constraints of the prevailing social and political climate.

HEALTHY BEHAVIOUR: PROMOTING POPULATION BEHAVIOUR CHANGE

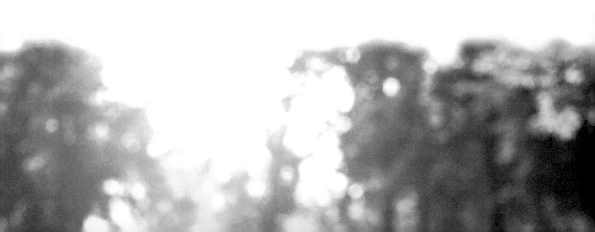

> The future health of millions of children, the sustainability of the NHS, and the eco-nomic prosperity of Britain all now depend on a radical upgrade in prevention and public health. Twelve years ago Derek Wanless' health review warned that unless the country took prevention seriously we would be faced with a sharply rising burden of avoidable illness. That warning has not been heeded – and the NHS is on the hook for the consequences.
>
> **NHS England, *Five Year Forward View*[26]**

People's health is to a large degree socially and behaviourally determined. The chances of a long and healthy life are influenced by circumstances such as a high-quality education, a good job, a secure and pleasant place to live with opportunities for participating in social and other activities that are important. Improving population health involves creating the social environment in which people can flourish, changing culture so that what is socially 'the norm' is also health promoting, and providing support for those who want to adopt healthier behaviours but struggle to do so. The social sciences have made considerable advances in discovering how to achieve this but it remains the case that many health interventions fail to achieve their goals, and interventions that might succeed fail to be adequately implemented. The former arises from limitations in the science and the latter arises partly from a failure of processes for translation into real-world contexts.

Following the publication of the *Five Year Forward View*, Sir Simon Stevens, Chief Executive of NHS England, made a series of speeches calling for concerted action on health promotion, noting that, despite increases in life expectancy, smoking still explains half the inequality in life expectancy between rich and poor, that binge drinking costs at least £5 billion a year in A&E admissions, road accidents, and extra policing, and that poor diets and insufficient physical activity are being 'normalised' along with obesity, which is increasing even among children.[27] Tackling these and similar issues requires more than new ways of delivering NHS services: population-wide measures of behavioural change will also be essential.[28]

Strikingly, we spend far less on research into prevention, health promotion and on how health services are delivered than we do on biomedical research. As the Academy of Medical Sciences notes, although the proportion spent on prevention has increased in recent years, it is still only about 5 per cent of the total spending on health research.

> Of the research funding spent on understanding causes of disease, only 20% is attributed to studying the environmental, psychological, social and economic factors, while the remaining 80% funds research into biological and endogenous factors. This has led to a number of specific evidence gaps and a lack of research capacity in key areas relevant to the health of the public.[29]

To illustrate, a US study in 2014 showed that funding for areas including the specific words 'gene', 'genome' or 'genetic' was 50 per cent greater than for areas including the more generally applicable word 'prevention'.[30]

Just one example of the cost of failing to take account of social and behavioural sciences was the enormous UK investment in vaccines in the 2009 influenza pandemic which were not taken up as planned because factors influencing behaviour were not sufficiently recognised or addressed.[31]

The most effective behavioural interventions are those that target multiple levels simultaneously and consistently,[32] reflecting the fact that behaviour is maintained by complex systems and can only be changed by disrupting those systems. Where this approach has been taken up, it has reaped dividends, as with England's Comprehensive Tobacco Control Plan, which was developed over years of close interaction between Government and social and behavioural experts in the area. Such examples of good practice are rare but could be increased with structures set up to enable social and behavioural scientists to work closely with policy-makers.

Resources are very often targeted at information campaigns, public health announcements or urging health providers to provide advice without considering the many other potentially more powerful drivers of behaviour and a scientific analysis of what is likely to be most effective. While information may make people more aware of the dangers of their behaviour, behaviour is more likely to change if there are also clear pathways to, and support for, change. This has been well established even in areas as complex as weight loss, where direction to weight loss programmes made a measurable difference.[33]

An example of behaviour change resulting from targeted support and widespread social intervention, halving of the rate of teenage pregnancies in England, arose in part from social science evidence about underlying social factors in teenage pregnancy. The evidence about the complex social causes of high teenage pregnancy rates resulted in a programme of interventions, led mainly by local government and schools, that resulted in this impressive decrease in the rate of teenage pregnancies.[34]

Teenage pregnancy: Success through joined up strategy

At the end of the twentieth century, the UK had the highest rate of teenage pregnancy in Western Europe.[35] Evidence about why UK teenagers were more likely to get pregnant informed the Government's 10-year Teenage Pregnancy Strategy for England in 1999: a complex, systems-based approach to prevention, including high-quality 'sex and relationships' education, youth-friendly contraceptive services, support for young parents to take part in education, employment and training, and programmes designed to change social norms.[36]

By 2013, the rate of teenage pregnancy had halved. The biggest reductions were seen in areas of highest deprivation where additional resources had been concentrated by the strategy. These successes were attributable to a long-term, multi-faceted intervention strategy. The strategy was also cost-effective: prevention of each teenage birth cost less than a quarter of the estimated additional cost of welfare support for such a birth.[37]

The funding for implementation was stopped after the 2010 General Election, despite the strategy's effectiveness, and further work is still needed to bring the UK's rate of teenage pregnancy in line with other high-income countries.[38]

The more established the behaviour, the greater the need to target fundamental mechanisms using a theoretically-informed and evidence-based analysis of the problem. The teenage pregnancy case study illustrates the need to bring together a clear conceptualisation of issues, using a range of methods. The underpinning research included 'real-world' longitudinal studies and qualitative methods to understand mechanisms of change, as well as large-scale pilot studies.

Policy-makers often rely heavily on common sense when making decisions instead of making use of available evidence from social and behavioural sciences. This has led to repeated policy failures and considerable unnecessary waste in resources and opportunities.

Part of the reason that more attention and resources are not devoted to enabling changes in behaviours and practices may be that we all 'do' behaviour, so it often appears that understanding human behaviour is 'obvious' and that it can be changed by the application of common sense.

MOT health checks: Assessing effectiveness through social science evidence

An example of wasted resources arising from insufficient use of findings from the social sciences is England's comprehensive annual NHS Health Checks, primarily being used to screen for cardiovascular risk factors.[39] Common sense may lead to the view that these would promote health and ultimately save money, because they can identify risk factors that can then be addressed. However, failing to take account of factors that influence the uptake of these checks, and the behaviour change that may arise from them, has severely limited their impact such that a recent analysis in the *BMJ* concluded that the funds would have been far better spent in other ways.[40]

What is needed is a more systematic investigation of the cost and efficacy of such interventions, so that promising preventative and health-promoting interventions can be prioritised, outcomes measured and widespread implementation put into place.

To do this, we need first to identify the key behaviours that need to change to achieve desired health improvements. But we also need a more comprehensive approach to considering the system of behaviours within and across individuals and their relationships with the social and material environments in which they occur. We also need a more comprehensive approach to the range of interventions that may be needed. While there may be a clear sense of the behaviours that need to change to produce desirable health outcomes, it is often the case that seemingly straightforward interventions are designed without considering a full repertoire of possible ways that behaviour change might be initiated or supported.

For instance, techniques labelled under the 'nudge' rubric that deploy some general findings from the study of human psychology – for instance, discounting the future in favour of the present or altering the choices that are easy for people to make so that they lead to better outcomes – are often popular among policy-makers because they seem less intrusive than other methods of influencing behaviour (such as regulation, pricing, taxing, and so on).[41] However, this misses strategies that are known to be effective at population level and to reduce inequalities, a point powerfully made in the 'intervention ladder' put forward in the 2007 report on public health by the Nuffield Council of Bioethics (see Figure 2).[42]

Figure 2   Ladder of intervention

Eliminate choice. Regulate in such a way as to entirely eliminate choice, for example through compulsory isolation of patients with infectious diseases.

Restrict choice. Regulate in such a way as to restrict the options available to people with the aim of protecting them, for example removing unhealthy ingredients from foods, or unhealthy foods from shops or restaurants.

Guide choice through disincentives. Fiscal and other disincentives can be put in place to influence people not to pursue certain activities, for example through taxes on cigarettes, or by discouraging the use of cars in inner cities through charging schemes or limitations of parking spaces.

Guide choices through incentives. Regulations can be offered that guide choices by fiscal and other incentives, for example offering tax-breaks for the purchase of bicycles that are used as a means of travelling to work.

Guide choices through changing the default policy. For example, in a restaurant instead of providing chips as a standard side dish (with healthier options available), menus could be changed to provide a more healthy option as standard (with chips as an option available).

Enable choice. Enable individuals to change their behaviours, for example by offering participation in an NHS 'stop smoking' programme, building cycle lanes, or providing free fruit in schools.

Provide information. Inform and educate the public, for example as part of campaigns to encourage people to walk more or eat five portions of fruit and vegetables per day.

Do nothing or simply monitor the current situation.

Source: Nuffield Council on Bioethics[43]

Politicians often favour 'nudges' and education campaigns over more effective policies because they are easy to implement, intuitive and do not conflict with vested interests or with strong personal beliefs about autonomy.

Part of the reason that focusing only on 'nudges' may appeal to policy-makers is that such interventions tend to focus on change by individuals and do not require more challenging social-structural changes which may yield larger benefits (by changing the social defaults of behaviour and reducing health inequalities) but require long-term commitment, often tackling powerful interests along the way.[44] Both theory and evidence show that policy changes aimed at altering the framework within which individuals make choices, sometimes restricting choices (such as not to wear seat belts), are powerful contributors to population health.

In the area of tax and benefit policy, the Institute of Fiscal Studies (IFS) has shown just how restricted the repertoire of policies is if only nudge or educational information-based policies are used.[45] The IFS argues that taking account of the full range of policy options is helpful when it is difficult for individuals to make 'rational' choices. For instance, where benefits are distant relative to the costs – as it is with eating healthy foods – the IFS report concludes that behavioural economics suggests there is a clearer rationale for using taxes or regulation to change consumption patterns than would be suggested by conventional economic models which tend to assume human behaviour is based on rational choice.[46] The need to consider the full range of interventions to bring about behaviour change is also stressed in the House of Lords report on behaviour change.[47]

The difficulties of introducing more intrusive fiscal interventions to improve health are demonstrated by the differing responses in Scotland and England and Wales to proposals for minimum alcohol unit pricing. The UK Government abandoned plans to introduce a minimum price per unit of alcohol in 2013; currently (spring 2017) the Scottish Government plans to introduce minimum unit pricing if it successfully sees off legal challenges. A recent review of the evidence by Public Health England concludes that minimum unit pricing of alcohol would make a significant contribution to population health, and would have particular benefits in reducing consumption among younger people.[48] This work was powerfully informed by much social and economic research, much of it led by the Interdisciplinary Alcohol Research Programme (IARP) at the University of Sheffield, involving social scientists from a number of institutions.[49]

Population behaviour change is greatest when a range of mutually supporting policy measures is combined with population health campaigns and provision of support for change.

Greatest benefits to health are likely to result when social structural changes are combined with more targeted interventions.[50] For example, in the case of tobacco control, raising tobacco taxes has clearly played an important role but when it was used as the only tobacco control measure in the 1990s there was no corresponding reduction in prevalence.[51] The ban on smoking in indoor public spaces has been a huge success in protecting the health of non-smokers, but its effect on smoking prevalence remains uncertain.[52] Social marketing campaigns, including No Smoking Day and Stoptober, have shown good evidence of being effective and highly cost-effective.[53] Targeted clinical interventions, in the form of brief opportunistic advice from physicians and provision of stop-smoking support, have led to a substantial increase in quitting.[54]

Brief advice: Untapped potential for smoking cessation

There are more than 40 high-quality randomised controlled trials showing that brief advice to smokers, given opportunistically during routine consultations, increases smoking cessation rates in patients.[55] This has been found to be one of the most cost-effective clinical interventions available to any health service in terms of cost per life year gained,[56] and there is no evidence that this effect has diminished over time.[57] The offer of a prescription or behavioural support increases the effectiveness of this intervention.[58]

On the basis of this evidence, GPs in England are given a financial incentive to provide brief advice and offer support for quitting, amounting to approximately £80 million each year. Unfortunately, while GP records report that such advice is given to more than 80 per cent of smokers, according to smokers the figure is more like 25 per cent.[59] Moreover, the introduction of the incentives did not increase the rate of prescribing stop-smoking medications.[60]

This is a key example of how social and behavioural science has been used to conceive an important public health intervention, but has not been used when considering how to implement it, with a huge opportunity cost and waste of public resources.

UNDERSTANDING BEHAVIOUR CHANGE

Behaviour occurs within a particular context and is influenced by factors interacting in complex ways. 'Systems thinking' is therefore necessary to understand and explain behaviour sufficiently to inform how to change it and maintain that change.[61] A clear map of the system within which one is trying to bring about change will inform decisions about where and how to intervene.[62]

Drawing on work of behavioural scientists, it is clear that there are three general areas that interventions *need to* target to change behaviour: people's capability (including having the necessary knowledge and skills); their motivation (including habits, emotional responses and analytic decision-making); and their opportunities (including the social and physical environments they face). The 'COM-B' (Capability Opportunity Motivation Behaviour) model helps direct attention to different mechanisms that might need to be addressed if health-related behaviours are to change (see Figure 3).[63]

Figure 3   The COM-B system

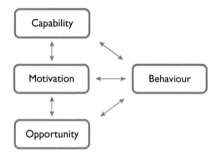

Source: Michie et al.[64]

COM-B forms the hub of a framework that was developed from a synthesis of 19 frameworks of behaviour change, the Behaviour Change Wheel. Around the hub are nine well-defined sets of possible interventions and seven policy domains in the outer wheel (see Figure 4).

It has been used by policy-makers to analyse their current policies to identify whether there are things missing and, if so, whether this is for a good reason, and it is also frequently used for designing behavioural interventions and policies. Because the selection of interventions and policies are based on an analysis of what needs to change, the framework enables the selection of interventions and policies that are likely to be effective. This also reminds us that achieving the goal of individual behaviour change may not always or most effectively rest on individual-level interventions: it often requires a number of systemic changes as well as strategies aimed at individuals and will usually be more successful if multiple levels support one another.

CAMPAIGN *for* SOCIAL SCIENCE

Table I Definitions of interventions and policies

Interventions	Definition	Examples
Education	Increasing knowledge or understanding	Providing information to promote healthy eating
Persuasion	Using communication to induce positive or negative feelings or stimulate action	Using imagery to motivate increases in physical activity
Incentivisation	Creating expectation of reward	Using prize draws to induce attempts to stop smoking
Coercion	Creating expectation of punishment or cost	Raising the financial cost to reduce excessive alcohol consumption
Training	Imparting skills	Advanced driver training to increase safe driving
Restriction	Using rules to reduce the opportunity to engage in the target behaviour (or to increase the target behaviour by reducing the opportunity to engage in competing behaviours)	Prohibiting sales of solvents to people under 18 to reduce use for intoxication
Environmental restructuring	Changing the physical or social context	Providing on-screen prompts for GPs to ask about smoking behaviour
Modelling	Providing an example for people to aspire to or imitate	Using TV drama scenes involving safe-sex practices to increase condom use
Enablement	Increasing means/reducing barriers to increase capability or opportunity[1]	Behavioural support for smoking cessation, medication for cognitive deficits, surgery to reduce obesity, prostheses to promote physical activity

Policies		
Communication/marketing	Using print, electronic, telephonic or broadcast media	Conducting mass media campaigns
Guidelines	Creating documents that recommend or mandate practice. This includes all changes to service provision	Producing and disseminating treatment protocols
Fiscal	Using the tax system to reduce or increase the financial cost	Increasing duty or increasing anti-smuggling activities
Regulation	Establishing rules or principles of behaviour or practice	Establishing voluntary agreements on advertising
Legislation	Making or changing laws	Prohibiting sale or use
Environmental/social planning	Designing and/or controlling the physical or social environment	Using town planning
Service provision	Delivering a service	Establishing support services in workplaces, communities etc.

[1]Capability beyond education and training; opportunity beyond environmental restructuring

Source: Michie *et al.*

Figure 4   The Behaviour Change Wheel

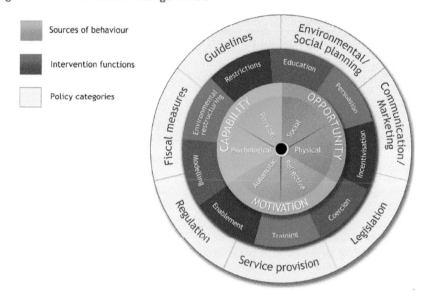

Source: The Behaviour Change Wheel: A Guide to Designing Interventions[65]

The Behavioural Insights Team and Nesta draw on a simplified version of this taxonomy in their EAST framework, aimed at making behavioural change 'Easy, Attractive, Social and Timely'.[66] But this framework does not draw attention to the range of policy interventions that may be useful in bringing about change, especially those that are not directed solely at individuals, and it does not link interventions to a theoretical model of behaviour.

STRATEGIES TO ENCOURAGE AND SUPPORT CHANGES IN HEALTH-RELATED BEHAVIOURS

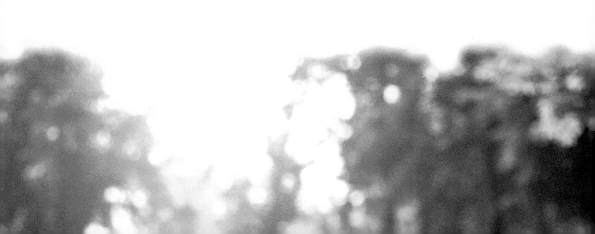

Strategies to support behaviour change may range from those targeted at individuals – for example, increasing numbers of smartphone apps and wearables to support behaviour change or individual 'treatment plans' – to enabling social support, changing environments that influence behaviour, changing services provided by local government, changing fiscal and regulatory frameworks and social policy interventions.

There is wide debate about the value and efficacy of health-based interventions that target individual behaviour and those that focus on community and cultural values. For example, there is a strong case for community-led participatory health research producing more enduring results, especially where communities are empowered to take control of factors that affect health outcomes, and so reduce inequalities in health.[67]

An example of an environmental strategy is the NHS Healthy New Towns programme that is working with ten housing developments to rethink how health and care services can be delivered by improving health through the built environment. The aim is to experiment in methods to support these new communities to 'design in' integrated local health and care services, and how they build in social and physical environments that improve health.[68]

Ambitious as this is, only a small proportion of the population lives in communities designed in this way. It will be an even greater challenge to consider how to encourage behaviour change in existing cities, towns and villages to increase physical activity. But drawing on a broad conceptual framework, such as the Behaviour Change Wheel, helps us consider the full range of options likely to be needed.

This sort of systems approach helped inform the Foresight report on obesity, with its system map for looking at causes of obesity and a range of interventions that go far beyond dietary advice.[69] But we are still a long way from designing a programme of evidence-based interventions that match the ambitions of the framework in the Foresight report, encompassing individual approaches, community behaviours and norms, changes in physical environments, and wide-ranging policy supports, including taxation and regulation. For example, there is growing evidence (despite claims from commercial vested interests) for the effectiveness of sugar taxes in reducing consumption of sugar-sweetened beverages.[70]

There are population-wide education campaigns led by Government and the Department of Health and others that provide information about the need for dietary and other changes to reduce cancer and heart disease.[71] We also have a growing number of 'meta-reviews' of evidence on various topics.[72] But there is less *accumulation* of evidence and experiment than there should and could be – and much less willingness to make the systemic multi-level change that will genuinely change population health.

For instance, it is acknowledged that information technology has great potential to improve people's ability to manage their own behaviours, but in evaluations of the effectiveness of wearable fitness trackers, for example, researchers have found these technologies did not on their own lead to weight loss.[73] Given the challenges of the size of sustained population change to tackle such issues as obesity or physical activity levels (both of which are important contributors to a number of acute and chronic health conditions), the UK needs to be committed to a more strategic focus on generating research, especially evaluations of interventions, to address these issues. Recent research providing international benchmarks on children's activity levels shows just what a large change in population behaviour would be needed to ensure healthy activity levels across the range of domains studied.[74]

SELF-MANAGEMENT OF ILLNESS AND LONG-TERM CONDITIONS

So far we have been considering strategies for preventing ill-health and promoting health and wellbeing among the general population and particular at-risk groups. However, as behaviour-related illnesses increase and the population ages, there has been a rapid increase in those with long-term health conditions. These require management by healthcare services, the people themselves and partnerships between those with long-term conditions and health and social care professionals.

According to the House of Commons Health Committee:

> Effective management of long-term conditions (LTCs) is widely recognised to be one of the greatest challenges facing the 21st-century National Health Service. ... Thanks to advances in the care and treatment of many common long-term conditions, a greater proportion of the population is now able to lead a longer and more active life: but this care and treatment consumes a greater proportion of the NHS's finite resources. 70% of total expenditure on health and care in England is associated with the treatment of the 30% of the population with one LTC or more, and the number of people in England with one or more such condition—currently 15 million—is projected to increase to around 18 million by 2025. Care for LTCs presently accounts for 55% of GP appointments, 68% of outpatient and A&E appointments and 77% of inpatient bed days. Cost pressures on the health and care system deriving from management of LTCs and treatment of the increasing prevalence of comorbidities is likely to add £5 billion to the annual costs of the system between 2011 and 2018.[75]

The effective management of long-term conditions requires patterns of behaviour by patients and healthcare providers that are different from the management of acute short-term conditions. Social and behavioural sciences are contributing to developing strategies to enhance patient engagement with self-management and biomedical and technological interventions, and to develop skills to achieve this. For example, where the management of the condition requires doing something counter-intuitive (for instance, exercising for lower back pain or arthritis). Techniques have been developed to initiate and maintain change over the long term. In addition, the social sciences can develop strategies to enhance quality of life, reduce disability and change behaviour to improve outcomes of chronic conditions or illnesses.

Figure 5 Care and treatment of long-term conditions in England

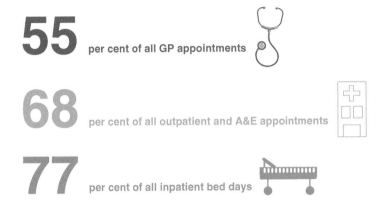

Care for people with LTCs account for:

55 per cent of all GP appointments

68 per cent of all outpatient and A&E appointments

77 per cent of all inpatient bed days

The 30 per cent of the population with LTCs accounts for 70 per cent of the health spend in England

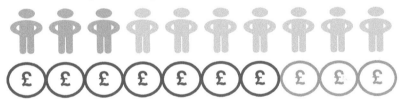

Effective support for managing long-term conditions requires a strategic and committed focus to join up systems of health and social care and support – delivered by healthcare professionals, a variety of officers and staff in local government, charities and peer supporters. Social science can help bridge the many gaps between agencies and pockets of good practice by focusing attention on the way social institutions can be brought together to produce better health outcomes and by bringing frameworks, methods and empirical findings from the social and behavioural sciences to bear on achieving this.

This is likely to be increasingly true as focus turns to technologies as an aid to health. There are a variety of increasingly accurate and affordable methods of support from new technologies, including smartphone apps, sensory and monitoring devices, internet-based programmes for sharing information and physiological and environmental sensors.[83] However, it is important to recognise that the use of such technologies are embedded in social relationships and practices, and their adoption and effective, sustained use depend on user engagement and application.[84]

These in turn depend on functions of the technology such as its personalisation, interactivity and responsivity as well as the user's social, political and cultural context, as research on the effectiveness of HIV prevention technologies has shown.[85] Technology design for behaviour change therefore requires a multi-disciplinary and multi-faceted approach.

Technology alone will not be sufficient to transform how people manage their health-related behaviours or how patients work with healthcare providers to manage long-term conditions. We need to recognise the diverse ways in which different people wish to use the technologies available and the extent to which they want to harness and integrate social support or work with their GPs or specialists. Social and behavioural scientists study how humans interact with technologies, the reasons for poor engagement and/or application,[86] and the development of strategies to enhance both engagement with such technologies and adherence to interventions within them. There is increasing evidence about how partnership-working with healthcare professionals and organisations can amplify the effect of digital interventions for managing long-term conditions.

— CASE STUDY —

Life after stroke: Using theory-based methods to reduce disability

An intervention has been developed based on a programme of research showing that, following stroke, people who believed that they had control over their recovery and outcomes were disabled to a lesser degree than people with similar impairments but lower confidence in their ability to control outcomes. The intervention uses recognised theory-based methods of enhancing self-efficacy delivered by a trained provider using the Stroke Workbook. It resulted in reduced disability at six months. The Stroke Workbook programme has been incorporated into Scottish Government guidelines.[76]

The stroke programme is managed by the same team that delivers the Heart Manual programmes,[77] which were developed based on evidence that these cognitive-behavioural interventions could improve quality of life following heart attacks and reduce the need for open-heart surgery. Other behavioural programmes have demonstrated that quality of life can be improved not only for the patients, but for their partners; one year after the intervention both patients and partners were less anxious and depressed as well as being more satisfied with the care they had received compared with a control group and these effects persisted to one year after the patients' heart attacks.[78]

Diabetes self-management: Improved outcomes through peer support

Nesta's Centre for Social Action Innovation Fund[79] has funded work to bring a promising social science-based intervention to improve the self-management of those with Type 2 diabetes. A large randomised controlled trial of a peer support model for diabetes has been carried out at Addenbrooke's Hospital. This combined peer group sessions with input from specialist nurses and trained volunteers to support diabetes patients to manage their conditions more effectively.[80] The results showed significant improvements in clinical outcomes, including physical measures such as blood pressure. Diabetes UK, the UK's largest charity for people with diabetes, plans to roll this model out nationally.

In addition, a joint commitment by NHS England, Public Health England and Diabetes UK has incorporated behavioural science in its own Diabetes Prevention Programme, Healthier You, aimed at those with a high risk of becoming diabetic. This programme provides tailored, personalised help to reduce the risk of Type 2 diabetes, including education on healthy eating and lifestyle, help to lose weight, bespoke physical exercise programmes and some social support. Following evidence that this reduces the risk of developing diabetes, further demonstration programmes are planned.[81]

In order to maintain behaviour change over time, long-standing routines and habits must change and new ones built into everyday life; peer group support has been one effective means of achieving this.[82]

BEHAVIOUR CHANGE AND IMPLICATIONS FOR HEALTH SERVICE DELIVERY

Social science research already plays an important role in helping to inform policy and practice about how health services are delivered. For example, economists, sociologists and others provide information about how UK health service delivery compares with other countries.[87] Social scientists provide independent information about medical careers and how to plan to ensure we have the healthcare workers we need in various settings, an issue of particular importance for the long-term prospects of the NHS.[88]

Planning for health services is a complex mix of patient needs and expectations – the 'demand' for services – and the way institutions and individuals work to deliver healthcare – the 'supply' side. Particular challenges facing healthcare systems include: variations in the delivery of healthcare, so that not all patients receive optimal care; the uncertain success of strategies to improve the delivery of care; and patchiness in the evidence needed to understand where improvements might be most important. Not only can the social sciences help understand these, but they can also help design experimental and quasi-experimental evaluations and time-series analysis to inform improved delivery for better patient outcomes.

Increasingly, it is clear that thoroughgoing organisational changes in the health services will be needed to implement measures that protect patients (for instance, to reduce hospital-induced infections) and to change clinical behaviour (for instance, prescribing behaviour) and managers' and commissioners' behaviours. Such changes also need to take account of the behaviours of patients whose expectations may need to be addressed (for example, if they expect antibiotics even when they are not an appropriate treatment).

Organisational change is dependent on a myriad of interdependent systems of human behaviours within the organisation. Change is often hard to achieve, not least because organisations are complex cultures, requiring not only strategic decisions but behavioural change at various levels to implement these decisions. Trade-offs of various sorts given competing resources (for example, time, money) and motivations (for example, professional identities, anxiety) are needed and social sciences can contribute in considering how best to balance the diverse needs and targets.

The case study shows that it was important to take seriously social science as *description* – asking what is going on; social science as *explanation* – understanding what interventions may work or what causes change in this setting; and social science as helping inform *implementation* and *generalisation*. Randomised trials may help us understand what interventions can work in certain contexts, but we need a richer mix of methods and frameworks or theories to guide successful, system-wide behaviour change.

Hospital checklists: Why the social matters

A recent example of how social sciences have helped drive behavioural change in healthcare delivery is the introduction of 'checklists' for various hospital procedures. Initially devised for intensive care, they aim to ensure that all essential steps are taken to reduce infection rates. The introduction of this simple procedure has the potential to have a significant impact on infection rates in hospitals.[89]

Studies of the implementation of checklists have found that a key element in the successful introduction of checklists rests on a social adaptive, not technical, change. That is, for such innovations in behaviour to take root, it is not enough to produce guidelines and a rational justification for their introduction. To bring about change, those using innovations such as checklists need to be motivated and committed to consistently change their behaviour – that is, to implement the checklist fully and wholeheartedly, as part of their normal team-working, and to take collective responsibility for adherence.

Think about what introducing the 'checklist' requires. None of the steps is contentious in itself. Indeed, they are all steps that a surgical team should in any case take to reduce the risk of infection. But it means ensuring that the wherewithal (soaps, drapes, and so on) are easily available – a system change requiring management and system support – and they need adherence by *all* members of a hierarchical team (so that nurses, for instance, can voice concern if doctors have skipped a step).[90] So successfully implementing something as simple as a checklist means it cannot be treated as a mere bureaucratic nicety.

A research collaboration led by a doctor and sociologist sought to understand more about the implementation of the use of the checklist in intensive care units in the USA. They found that the reason the checklist worked in reducing rates of central venous catheter bloodstream infections in these intensive care units is that they changed the culture, including peer norms about the inevitability of infection, by developing a whole-team approach to safety.[91] Successive evaluations of implementing these checklists in the UK – where initially the dramatic results achieved elsewhere were not matched – showed the importance of understanding and using the social process of implementation.[92]

Although the items in the intensive care unit checklist are all standard procedures, providing the checklist in the way described hits all three key levers for behaviour change. Changing the **opportunities** (making it easier by having all the resources to hand), changing **capabilities** (enabling all members of the team to be engaged and take responsibility for the actions of others), and changing **motivation** (by showing that infections can be dramatically reduced) all play their part in bringing about change. Targeting capability, opportunity and motivation, as suggested by the COM-B model,[93] has also been shown to be effective in other healthcare interventions, for example increasing hand hygiene behaviours and reducing hospital acquired infections. Behavioural scientists were at the centre of developing an England-wide intervention to improve hand hygiene among nurses and evaluating it across 60 hospital wards in 16 hospitals, using a randomised 'stepped-wedge' evaluation design.[94] This is a rigorous and practical study design that can be used to evaluate services and practices when innovations are introduced, translating healthcare activity into generalisable evidence.[95]

The following case studies illustrate the importance of providing a range of interventions beyond providing information to change the behaviour of healthcare professionals.

A key feature of these studies is that while having data was a necessary condition for identifying where change in behaviour of health professionals might be needed, it was insufficient to produce behaviour change. Many funders of research on health service delivery now recognise the need to take a wider approach. For instance, the Health Foundation, in addition to funding Fellowships and PhDs in Improvement Science, is providing about £30 million over 10 years to support a research institute to develop and apply knowledge that has a direct and positive impact on health services. Prolonged investment is needed to ensure the two-way iteration between knowledge and the practical application that is necessary for advancing both science and its translation.

This is particularly important since a common-sense approach to changing practice is often to provide additional education or training. This has often been the case in relation to health professionals. An example where failure to change among health professionals was not due to lack of information (capability), but was due to lack of motivation and opportunity comes from the dental service in Scotland. A guideline for dentists on placing fissure sealants to protect children's teeth was only partially implemented and a trial was conducted to examine the benefits of further education and/or the reward of an additional fee for this service.[100] The education had no effect but the rewards increased the rate of compliance with the guidelines. The results had an immediate impact as the Chief Dental Officer incorporated the trialled intervention into the fee structure for dentists on the day the results were reported.

Prescribing patterns: Reducing variation through changing clinical behaviour

Variations in prescribing can result in unnecessary spending. There is variation in the rates with which GPs and hospital doctors prescribe branded, rather than generic, versions of statins, even when the evidence suggested the generic version would work as well, and save money. Working in a team with doctors and data analysts, a project made data to inform a prescribing practice available for GPs and other doctors on a website (Openprescribing.net).[96]

But simply having open data is not enough, welcome though it is (see new tools such as Podcast, an online resource to help in prescribing decisions).[97] In a collaboration between the Behavioural Insights Team, Public Health England, the Department of Health and others, data were used to identify GP practices that prescribed antibiotics at rates significantly higher than others in their area. The researchers then used a random assignment trial to test the effect of sending a letter to these practices telling them their rate of prescribing antibiotics was higher than 80 per cent of their peers. The results showed that the letter significantly reduced prescription rates. (A separate variant tested a letter telling GPs that over-prescription of antibiotics was not good for patients; this had no significant effect.) Information alone was not enough: it was important to motivate change by ensuring GPs compared themselves with peer practice.[98]

Tackling prescribing variations arising from departure from 'best practice' is not just a matter of saving money or protecting the population as a whole; prescription practices can cause harm. A team in Scotland designed a complex intervention aimed at reducing the number of patients who were inappropriately prescribed nonsteroidal anti-inflammatory drugs and antiplatelet medications that can cause gastrointestinal, cardiovascular and renal complications and hospital admissions. The intervention included professional education about balancing the risks and benefits of prescriptions, an initial financial incentive for reviewing high-risk patients, and a tool to make it easier to identify high-risk patients and to consider the options for them. Using the tool also required doctors to complete information about what they decided to do and why. The study showed significant reductions in prescribing patterns, even after the financial incentive stopped, and a wider impact on related emergency hospital admissions.[99]

Even such a simple goal as ensuring that all health workers wash their hands – an important part of reducing the spread of infections – is not consistently achieved. Improving this has benefitted from the development and evaluation of interventions using social and behavioural science.

CASE STUDY

Clean Your Hands: An effective intervention informed by theory

Although hand-washing is widely known to prevent the spread of infection in hospitals, compliance with clinical practice guidelines has been poor.

Many of the barriers are social. Significant factors have been shown to include the inaccessibility of sinks and alcohol rubs, forgetfulness, and deficiencies in the communication of good practice in infection control.[101]

A campaign, Clean Your Hands, was devised to increase health workers' hand-washing opportunities, by placing alcohol hand rub near beds, and motivation, through use of visual propaganda, one-to-one staff feedback mechanisms, and by encouraging patients to ask.[102]

Evaluation showed that soap and alcohol hand rub use – indicated by procurement – tripled, rates of MRSA and *C difficile* infection fell,[103] and feedback mechanisms made staff 13–18 per cent more likely to wash their hands.[104]

Further research has been commissioned by the Health Foundation to examine the effect of 'micro-environmental' interventions – citrus smells and images like watching eyes – on hand-washing practice.[105]

SOCIAL SCIENCE AND NEW WAYS OF CONFIGURING SERVICES

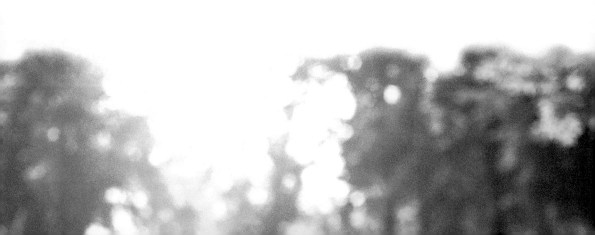

So far we have been looking at changing the behaviours of health professionals and illustrated some of the ways in which the social sciences have contributed. But there are also system-level changes for which robust social science evidence could make a difference.[106] While the translation of organisational change into improved health is mediated by changes in individual behaviour, it is important to understand how changes in social settings work at multiple levels. This can inform the types of organisational change, such as incentive structures and opportunities for those behaviour changes, which can alter the behaviour of health professionals. Behaviour is not only relevant as a mediator; it is often a key part of the organisational intervention itself, for example, in improving communication and team-working.

The ways in which health services are delivered in the UK are increasingly recognised to be key to improving population health. Partly this is a result of financial pressures and the drive for efficiency, and partly it is because the UK's ratio of doctors to the population is low relative to EU comparators.[107] Approaches suggested to improve service delivery include widening the responsibilities of the existing non-medical workforce,[108] addressing reasons for retirement and emigration of doctors,[109] changing recruitment numbers for particular medical specialities,[110] and the greater use of digital technologies (for example, Skype consultations). A programme of rigorous evaluation of new ways of delivering services is especially important given the rise in the proportion of the population with long-term health conditions, and with complex co-morbidities.

For many long-term conditions, we are a long way from having models of active and easy-to-attend services in community settings that promote a step change in patient behaviours and outcomes. Reconfiguring complex continuing services for chronic conditions will require a programme of focused work.

To improve healthcare delivery, regional NHS directorates have set up 'Vanguard' areas to experiment with new ways of configuring services. In Scotland, the Scottish Collaborative Innovation Partnership Process (SCIPP) examines some of the same issues. These include better integration of primary and acute care; enhanced healthcare within care homes; multi-speciality providers for common conditions within communities; and reconfiguration of urgent and emergency care. Some of these changes in healthcare delivery have been subject to some degree of piloting (setting up an experiment, and collecting objective evidence about operation and outcomes), such as the work of the Central London Clinical

Commissioning Group.[114] Social scientists have been involved in the design of each of these evaluations.[i]

Service reconfiguration: How social science insights inform best practice

NICE Guidelines spell out the health checks and services that newly diagnosed diabetics should get, and an NHS National Service Framework for Diabetes gives further guidance on what this should mean for service delivery. Yet the National Audit Office has found that the majority of diabetics are still not receiving all of the specified care processes, and fewer than 4 per cent of newly-diagnosed diabetes patients were recorded as having taken up a structured education programme.[111] This is not merely a question of individual behaviour but of how local services support those with new diagnoses to take up the programmes and those with longer-standing diagnoses to adopt the diet and other behavioural changes required to manage their condition. Integrated practice units for joined-up diabetes care are now being implemented, for example, in the inner-London borough of Camden.[112]

A successful reconfiguration of services has also taken place around the delivery of care to those who have recently had strokes. Research suggested that referring stroke patients directly to care in a specialist stroke unit that could provide immediate assessment by specialist teams, brain imaging and thrombolysis when appropriate, and acute rehabilitation services, was the single biggest factor that could improve outcomes after stroke, even if patients had to travel further to reach such units. In London, evidence based on statistical modelling and informed by a social science team, who considered a wide range of evidence about the importance of specialist care, was used to reconfigure patterns of provision to ensure that all patients could reach such units within 30 minutes and that only units providing care 24 hours a day, seven days a week would be used. In Manchester, a slightly different model was used, with units offering less comprehensive care also being used as a first port of call. In London, some units that were providing less comprehensive care were closed, while none were in Manchester. Analysis showed that deaths and length of hospital stays were reduced in London, while Manchester did not see a similar reduction in death rates.[113]

---

[i] These initiatives are different from the place-based NHS Sustainability and Transformation plans. While these involve reconfiguring services and changing ways of service delivery to integrate provision, they are driven in part by the need to seek cost efficiencies.

There are also already a number of initiatives to improve the links between services and research, including social science research,[115] such as the GP Access Fund for pilots to improve access, networks listed in the NHS Improvement Directory,[116] and the NHS Innovation Accelerator.[117]

Many but not all of these projects and programmes have involved evaluation and programmes for rolling them out more widely.[118] However, it is not clear that these initiatives add up to more than the sum of their parts – that there is a strategic setting of priorities, cumulative learning and attention to issues arising from implementation. Social science could be better used to evaluate pilots and devise implementations in an iterative manner. The Health Foundation's proposed Improvement Science Institute is one way to address this. More strategic 'implementation labs' would be another, as set out in the recommendations of this report.

The social and behavioural sciences have expertise in the study of and support for implementation across a range of services, including health, education and social services. Evidence has shown that successful implementation of interventions depends on social processes and interactions, and interventions cannot just be copied like a recipe book. What may work in one social setting or culture may not work in another. Understanding the reasons for this is vital in informing successful implementations in new settings. Changes in service delivery rest on a complex combination of institutional practices and cultures, incentives and regulatory changes. (See the journal *Implementation Science* for current evidence and thinking in this area.)[119] But using the theories, evidence and methods from the social sciences to greater effect in this arena means we need to have the right capacity for this type of work and ways of ensuring they are brought to bear in a focused way.

Implementation research is becoming a cornerstone even of behavioural economics with significant programmes of research devoted to understanding the relevant conditions for change for particular issues in particular settings, including incentives for change.[120] There are similar national and international initiatives in children's and education services.[121]

In a devolved healthcare system, with local healthcare Trusts and Commissioning Groups and different national ways of organising care, variation in ways of providing services will be normal and desirable. Using these variations to look at whether they may give rise to different outcomes can provide useful evidence for improvement.[122]

However, local experiments may not result in generalisable lessons or strategic focus, and will not in themselves provide cumulative learning about what changes may make the most difference. Understanding the settings and the conditions that affect complex interventions or reorganisations requires a range of evidence: understanding the ways in which people actually work, as well as understanding the ways in which opportunities and motivations may be changed in the routine working environments involving the whole range of staff (rather than the more highly-motivated staff who tend to participate in studies). Resources to pilot different ways of working should ideally be planned and reviewed with strategic attention, so that local pilots test key variables in ways that may allow generalisation.

Without this process of piloting and evaluation, we risk failing to exploit opportunities to enhance the effectiveness of existing ways of changing behaviour. For example, audit and feedback aims to improve patient care and outcomes through careful review of healthcare performance against explicit standards. It is widely used to monitor and improve NHS care, including in national clinical audit programmes. Audit and feedback is one of the more effective interventions to change health professional practice.[123] Cumulative meta-analysis of audit and feedback trials indicates that effect sizes stabilised over 10 years ago, suggesting a lack of cumulative learning on how to improve effectiveness.[124] There are opportunities to systematically embed audit and feedback trials within national clinical audit programmes as part of an ambitious international 'meta-laboratory'.[125]

The social sciences have much to offer here, both methodologically and in generating substantive hypotheses that can be tested. Only in this way can local, one-off experiments look beyond 'what works' in a single location to the question of how and why some service innovations work in some settings and not in others.[126]

None of these insights is new, of course, and variations in healthcare practices provide in themselves a fruitful field of inquiry. But there is growing recognition of the importance of social and behavioural science not only to help explain these variations but to help reduce them to improve healthcare practice. The time is right to move beyond considering these issues on a project-by-project basis and build a more robust infrastructure to propose, examine, evaluate and help promote social and organisational change in service delivery to improve the nation's health.

SOCIAL SCIENCE AND DATA

Policy organisations, such as the King's Fund, and research funders, such as the Wellcome Trust, the Health Foundation, the ESRC and MRC, along with health professionals and clinical and social scientists have been increasingly vocal in calling attention to the need for more strategic understanding of health – how outcomes relate both to the health services and to wider social and environmental factors – and have pointed out that this requires making better use of data.[127] So too have the Department of Health, NHS England and the Local Government Association, among others.[128]

For much social and healthcare research, data are analogous to the scientist's laboratory. This is recognised in initiatives such as the Health Foundation's research programme on health informatics, which funds projects and capacity to improve use of all sorts of routine data to improve healthcare.[129] The Academy of Medical Sciences report, *Improving the Health of the Public by 2040*, also draws attention to the need for better use of data, and the need to build the capacity of researchers from all disciplines to use those data.[130]

So while the issue of data underpins much of the substantive discussion in this report, it is important enough as an issue in its own right to warrant a separate discussion.

As we have argued above, appreciation that examining variations in healthcare can provide valuable insight has widened the drive to consider how routine health and administrative data can be a pathway to improving medical care. (The Dartmouth Institute in the US was one of the first research institutions to recognise this systematically.[131]) For instance, in its 2015 report, *Better Value in the NHS*, the King's Fund examined a range of ways that better value (with better outcomes and less spending) had been achieved by the NHS over a number of years, and pointed out that in one important area there was still much to be done. Writing about variations in care, the report says:

> The scale of these quality problems in the NHS is powerfully illustrated by data on the variations in clinical practice. These variations are widespread both within and across different parts of the country – so wide that they are not explained by differences in people's health needs and patients' preferences. In other words, these variations are unnecessary and avoidable.
>
> Why is there a more than 1,000-fold variation in the rate that GPs refer patients for some diagnostic tests? Why do rates of elective tonsillectomy in children range from 145 to 424 per 100,000 young people? Put more simply, why do some people in the NHS receive much better care than others? Answering these questions and tackling the resulting variations in care is one of the most significant ways for the NHS to improve quality and value.[132]

Understanding variations in healthcare by making better use of data is an important means to improving healthcare. Over the past decade or more, the NHS has made enormous strides in its use of data and statistics (though even in the case of national statistics discussions continue about how to improve statistical series further).[133]

Similar efforts are underway to improve the ability of the NHS to capture information in digital form so that they can be used in analyses that will improve healthcare. While GPs and others in primary care now largely work from digital records, hospitals are some way behind. In September 2016, the National Advisory Group on Health Information Technology in England – the Wachter review – published its findings on how the NHS should move forward to use information technology to produce better digital records for hospital-based care.[134] That review stresses the importance of having better data on hospital care as a means of improving healthcare and safety, noting that any cost savings will come later, not early on in the process. It also emphasises the importance of having such data for public health research, noting the gains to be made from hospitals sharing data about patients, while much research can use anonymised data.

> Patient information, collected through GP EHRs, has been used in public/private collaborations for research, epidemiological surveillance and quality improvement. As one example, the Clinical Practice Research Datalink (CPRD) extracts anonymised records from more than 600 practices for use in research studies and clinical trials. Specific cohorts of patients (i.e., those with kidney disease or with diabetes) can be created and examined for treatment patterns or clinical outcomes. Another project linked anonymised GP data on more than 2 million patients to national mortality data to create a well-validated cardiovascular risk algorithm (QRisk2). In other words, the potential to undertake such innovative work at a national scale and at minimal cost is already being realised for ambulatory practices, and would increase significantly once hospital records are also digitised.[135]

In other ways, there are better data on spending related to hospitals than there are for primary care. This variability hampers much work that economists and other social scientists could do to compare spending for different parts of the UK and compare it to outcomes, as well as allowing international comparisons. As the Institute for Fiscal Studies put it recently:

> Finally, the data available on medical spending in England are far less comprehensive than those for comparable countries in Europe, despite operating a national public health system. Information is restricted to hospital use, which constitutes less than half of NHS spending. The scrapping of the care.data programme, which sought to

bring together information from different health and social care settings, means that unfortunately this situation is unlikely to change in the near future. Moreover, maximising the use of hospital data that are available in England is hampered by restrictions on access and delays in linking to survey data, even when there is consent from individuals to do so. This places limitations on the extent to which patterns of individual-level spending and the links between costs and service provision in different parts of the health and social care system can be fully understood. The fact that data coverage and access are far more restricted in England than in many other countries reduces the amount of research carried out on the efficacy of healthcare delivery across the NHS, thereby making it harder to uncover possibilities for service improvement. Ultimately, patients may pay the price for this.[136]

For some purposes, using data to improve healthcare requires 'personal' data: data about individuals, their backgrounds and circumstances and about the care they receive. But much of the data needed for research is 'de-identified' (this is a legal and technical term). It is still data about individuals but removes names, addresses and many other personal identifiers. This distinction between health records and data that are personal and confidential and data that are 'de-identified'[137] is still the subject of much public discussion. The Caldicott *Review of Data Security, Consent and Opt-Outs* proposes steps to ensure data security and safeguards for privacy, including consent, for personally-identifiable health data.[138]

The Caldicott Review notes that de-identified data for research do not generally require consent, though data security and special safeguards during the stage when data are being stripped of personal identifiers remain essential. The report notes that 'the absence of such data, particularly from GP practices and social care, makes it difficult for commissioners to evaluate the impact of interventions across all care settings', citing a National Audit Report to the effect that 'the Department [of Health] and NHS England are taking steps to improve access but they are making decisions without fully understanding either the demand for services or the capacity of the current system. Given the important role general practice plays in the health and social care system, the Department and NHS England need better data in order to make well-informed decisions about how to use limited resources to best effect.'[139]

Social scientists and statisticians have long been aware of the importance of clear thinking about privacy and consent, even with regard to de-identified data. Over time they have evolved what might be called a 'social consent model' for research. This goes beyond thinking about the characteristics of the data themselves but also takes into account how data are used and reported, and other protections of privacy.

THE SOCIAL CONSENT MODEL

This model is based on five principles described by some as the 'five safes'.[140]

- Safe projects: Is the purpose of research for public benefit? It is important that decision-makers include lay people, not just other researchers, and that there is full transparency and public justification of what projects are funded.
- Safe people: Only trained and trusted researchers who agree to rules with clear enforcement mechanisms should have access to de-identified individual-level data.
- Safe settings: The data need to be held in settings with strong safeguards.
- Safe outputs: None of the results of analysis should identify (or seek to identify) anyone.
- Safe data: The data must be appropriate for the intended use, and contain only the sensitive or confidential information required for the purposes of the research.

This 'social consent' model has several important features. First, it does not focus solely on the characteristics of the data themselves. Different data sets may contain data of differing degrees of sensitivity, but the need for safe people, and secure settings and safe outputs means that there are other safeguards to protect privacy and prevent identification. Perhaps, however, the most important feature is that the research can only be done after a clear case is made that it is for public benefit, with lay people (people other than researchers or funders or policy-makers) involved in the decision. It is essential, too, that the projects be transparently undertaken. These features give rise to a social consent, with due attention to privacy and balancing public good and private rights.

Use of this model has been informed by social science research about the safeguards that the public expects for such work. In 2013 the ESRC and Office for National Statistics (ONS) commissioned a national survey on using administrative data for research. It asked people about their initial views and then provided information and discussion before asking for their views again.[141] This 'deliberative' model allows people to consider complicated issues without being led to a particular conclusion. Most people supported data-sharing with appropriate safeguards and a clear judgement about public benefit. In 2016 a national survey was conducted on commercial access to health data for public-benefit research.[142] Here the picture is more nuanced, with support for business access to health data only when there is clear public benefit. So we have robust social science evidence that the safeguards in this model respond to public concerns about privacy while also meeting their positive wish that data are used to improve population health.

The social consent model underpins the Administrative Data Research Network (ADRN), funded by the ESRC, to ensure that 'administrative data' – data routinely gathered by government as part of its normal work – can be used in research. This has involved setting up a considerable infrastructure for trusted third party matching of different data sets to be linked, ensuring strong security settings and, perhaps most importantly, ensuring independent assessment of the public benefit of any research proposed. One aim of the ADRN is to be able to link health data with social data (covering such issues as benefits and income, receipt of social care, local housing conditions, and so on) precisely so we can understand more about the relationships between health and social factors. This sort of data linkage is essential if we are to take a wide view of how to improve population health.

The largest UK initiative in 'health informatics' is the Farr Institute, supported by 10 funders, including the Medical Research Council, the Wellcome Trust and other medical research charities; the National Institute for Health Research, the Chief Scientist Office (Scotland) and the National Institute of Health and Social Care Research (Wales); and the ESRC and Engineering and Physical Sciences Research Council. Twenty-one universities and various other partners will conduct health research using clinical, environment and population data. They also have a remit to build research capacity, inform policy and engage with public debates about the use of data to improve public health.

Despite these two large-scale initiatives, and the infrastructure that meets public concerns, there are still many obstacles in the way of achieving the sort of access to health data that social scientists and others need to achieve the aspirations set out in this report. NHS Digital, which holds the health data needed for analyses (other than statistical aggregates), has been reluctant to grant access to individual-level 'de-identified' data, in part owing to the controversy over the now discontinued 'care.data' programme, the NHS England and Health and Social Care Information Centre programme designed to bring together health and social care information from different healthcare settings,[143] which was not set up with the same framework or safeguards as the ADRN.

Both the health research and social science communities are aware that they have much to do to work with the public to clarify the benefits and the risks of using data. The views of the public on the balance between individual privacy and common good are crucial to this process. Views on the appropriate balance will be different for different people, but we need a clear structure for considering when consent is essential (when data are personally identifiable), and when the social consent model is more appropriate. The Wellcome Trust has convened an initiative[144] to ensure the research community does better in explaining what is at stake and continues to use good evidence to engage with all those who want to understand why data are so important for the health of people.[i] Meanwhile, with the challenges facing the NHS, and the importance of using all available tools to address them, we need a renewed sense of urgency in unlocking the current impasse in providing data for public-benefit research.

[i]At the time of this report, both the Digital Economy Bill 2016-17 and a private member's Data Guardian Bill are before Parliament, and both may help to promote wider access. But much will depend on how NHS Digital and various government departments respond to opening up data to independent inquiry.

RECOMMENDATIONS

Social sciences have an important role in improving population health, by promoting healthy behaviours and the social changes that support these, better chronic disease self-management, and improvements in health professional practice and health service delivery. It could, under the right conditions, contribute much more. For that to happen, we need appropriate expertise, evidence that accumulates and has strategic focus, and evaluated iterations between innovations, evidence and implementation.

Figure 6 identifies the areas of action that are required in a new national strategy. These are elaborated in Table 2. A national strategy for social sciences and health needs to:

1. Identify key stakeholders and actors in the public sector, third sector and private sector.
2. Establish for each of the areas of activity in Figure 6 who is doing what, where the most promising areas for improvement are, and who should be responsible.
3. Construct a coherent plan for the short, medium and long term, specifying targets, evaluation methods and milestones.

The following recommendations are designed to provide the foundation for development of such a national strategy for maximising the impact of social sciences on the health of people.

1. RECOMMENDATIONS FOR COORDINATING AND FUNDING RESEARCH AND IMPLEMENTATION

There are already many collaborations and centres that are primarily based in social science academic settings but include projects and outreach with health specialists and practitioners. These include such examples as the five UK Clinical Research

Figure 6   Areas of activity required for a national strategy to improve the quality and impact of social and behavioural sciences in the area of population health

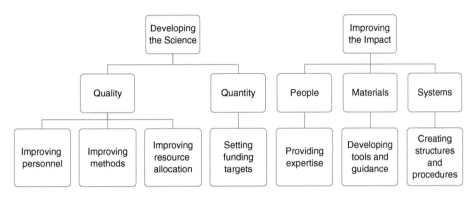

Table 2   Activities required in a new national strategy for social sciences and health

Improving personnel	Improved education and training of social scientists and key users of social science in health and social care
Improving methods	Development of more advanced methods for generating and testing models and theories, and for developing and evaluating interventions; includes use of machine learning and advanced statistical techniques to capitalise on large and complex data sets
Improving resource allocation	More systematic processes for rational allocation in research funding, applying social science understanding to these processes taking account of what is known about bias and error in human judgement; adoption of efficient systems for evaluation of funding strategies and their implementation
Setting funding targets	Using social science understanding to establish practicable and acceptable methods for increasing the funding for social sciences in the context of competing priorities and interests
Providing expertise	Creating roles and responsibilities within stakeholder and user organisations for the translation of social science findings into policy and practice
Developing tools and guidance	Developing tools and guidance to improve capability to determine policies and practices most likely to meet the 'APEASE' criteria of Affordability, Practicability, Effectiveness, Acceptability, Safety, and Equity; this includes online decision support based on social science
Creating structures and procedures	Put in place structures and procedures to embed social science findings, methods and expertise in policy-making and practice within local and central government and other key organisations

Collaboration (UKCRC) Public Health Research Centres of Excellence;[145] the Health Protection Research Units (HPRUs), which are research partnerships between universities and Public Health England;[146] the Behaviour and Health Research Unit at the University of Cambridge;[147] the National Prevention Research Initiative;[148] the University College London (UCL) Centre for Behaviour Change;[149] and the soon-to-be announced Health Foundation-funded improvement research centre.[150]

These centres have varying roles and thematic approaches. Some have a strong academic focus, while others put more weight on engagement with practitioners and policy-makers. Some are funded solely by one funder, while others are (or were originally) funded as a collaboration between different funders. They cover a variety of research topics and together have made important contributions to the research and evidence available to improve health in the UK.

To these academically-based centres should be added various others, most notably two networks of centres in England funded by NHS England and the National Institute for Health Research.

The Academic Health Science Networks (AHSNs) were established by NHS England in 2013 to spread innovation to improve health at pace and scale. The creation of AHSNs was recommended in Sir David Nicholson's December 2011 report *Innovation, Health and Wealth*,[151] which identified the need to improve patient and population health outcomes by translating research into practice and building a stronger relationship with the scientific and academic communities and industry. Each AHSN centre works across a distinct geography serving a different population in each region, and also comes together to promote joint learning and the wider adoption of promising innovation across all areas.

The challenges facing the AHSNs require medium- and long-term activities, and building relationships within each geographic area and the AHSNS themselves are relatively young.[152]

The National Institute for Health Research has funded 13 Collaborations for Leadership in Applied Health Research and Care (CLAHRCs) to undertake high-quality applied health research focused on the needs of patients and to support the translation of research evidence into practice in the NHS. CLAHRCs are collaborative partnerships between a university and the surrounding NHS organisations, focused on improving patient outcomes through the conduct and application of applied health research. They create and embed approaches to research and its dissemination that are specifically designed to take account of the way that healthcare is increasingly delivered across sectors and across a wide geographical area.

These centres therefore have a range of remits, some mainly geographically based and focused on creating networks of academics and practitioners, while others have a more substantive thematic focus. But we need a more strategic focus if we are to take forward a preventative, health-promoting agenda for change.

Recommendation 1.1

We call for a UK strategic coordinating body for research into population health. It should bring together major research funders (such as National Institute for Health Research (NIHR), Medical Research Council (MRC), the Economic and Social Research Council (ESRC), Wellcome Trust, Cancer Research UK, and British Heart Foundation), public health bodies (such as Public Health England, Health Protection Scotland, Public Health Wales, Public Health Agency for Northern Ireland, NHS England, Scotland, Wales and Northern Ireland), and relevant learned societies (such as the Academy of Social Sciences and Academy of Medical Sciences).[153]

Recommendation 1.2

We recommend that this coordinating body should take as its remit a wide view of population health, and approaches to improving it, recognising (i) the role of behaviour in improving health and the environmental and social systems within which behaviour occurs and changes, and (ii) the diversity of change agents at population, community and individual level influencing health indirectly as well as directly. Its aim should be to support high-quality, multi-disciplinary research on these issues and on how best to translate research evidence into policy and practice. In deliberating about how to improve population health through research, we believe that not only must funders act more strategically, but they must also consider how to ensure that the research itself is strategic. That means it should provide for longer-term programmes of work rather than simply a range of one-off projects, and should have a clear remit to include not only research into promising innovations and interventions – to understand what interventions might work in population or patient behaviour change, or in health professional behaviour change or service delivery reconfiguration – but also to consider the capacity for larger-scale piloting and implementation strategies.

Recommendation 1.3

One of the new body's first tasks should be to commission a review of the existing infrastructure for social and behavioural research and its implementation in healthcare and public health, involving stakeholders, funders, and major research centres. This review should examine research funding, funding agencies, funding mechanisms, and infrastructure for implementation at national, regional and local level, including resources and roles dedicated to this.

Recommendation 1.4

In addition to coordinating funding, the review should make recommendations regarding the building of an integrated system for multi-disciplinary research and implementation. This would include reviewing existing centres and networks, addressing the weaknesses in the current approaches while building on their strengths, to ensure critical mass and stability. This should include centres that provide interdisciplinary national substantive expertise – involving social and biomedical sciences – as well as those that attempt to provide regionally-based translational networks. The aim should be to ensure coverage of all important topics to do with population health, important groups of patients at risk of or who have chronic conditions where behavioural change is important, but should also include service delivery innovations.

In mapping existing centres it seems clear that we need not only coordination in funding, but in devising ways in which networks of centres, both new and existing, can liaise more closely with one another.[154] New centres with thematic substantive focus on behaviour change will be one fruitful avenue to explore. We advocate central funding as this is the surest way to ensure researchers and practitioners are genuinely working together, which takes time, particularly if programmes of work are to be genuinely interdisciplinary, and move from experiment to implementation (the 10-year funding for the Health Foundation's new improvement institute is indicative of what may be needed). **It should include a focus on how to ensure that understanding and overcoming barriers to adoption of health service improvements are given sufficient importance.**

Part of the aim of the strategic funding body should be to move from a culture of one-off experiments to a structure that supports cumulative evidence about how to bring about change, and a sufficient engagement with NHS trusts as well as strategic practitioners and clinicians, to iterate between promising innovations and programmes of implementation. This will require support at the highest levels of the NHS, the Department of Health, Public Health England, and others.

We recommend that the review should consider establishing a number of 'implementation laboratories'. There are frequent failures to introduce effective new interventions and clinical practices quickly enough, and to consistently use those already proven to be effective, or to stop using those found to be ineffective or even harmful.[155] There is therefore a need for research, experiment and evaluation that examines how to improve the uptake of effective interventions. Implementation research aims to inform policy decisions about how best to use resources to improve the uptake of research findings by evaluating approaches to change professional and organisational behaviour.[156] This should include research into how to increase the speed of up take of research-based innovations, including those that involve new ways of working and service innovation. This will be particularly challenging at a time of pressure on NHS expenditure. The implementation laboratories should iterate between trials, evaluations and wider-scale implementation.

One possibility is that incentives for implementation could be built into existing audit and feedback, widely used to monitor and improve NHS care, including in national clinical audit programmes. Audit and feedback generally has small to moderate and variable effects.[157] Yet cumulative meta-analysis of audit and feedback trials indicates that effect sizes stabilised over 10 years ago, suggesting a lack of cumulative learning on how to improve effectiveness.[158]

In any case, focusing not just on the supply of evidence but on how to provide stronger systemic incentives for organisations within the NHS should be an urgent priority for strategic consideration by the new body coordinating health research. This presents an important agenda for new research.

If this agenda is adopted, we recommend that discussion should be widened to include not only research funders, but a range of other bodies with interests in innovation and behaviour change across a wide range of health interests. This should include those with direct interests in healthcare delivery (the NHS in each nation; Public Health England and its counterparts; local government; strategic health researchers; and social scientists in universities and in bodies with an existing programme of work (Nesta and the Behavioural Insights Team, for example)). Some of the issues to be considered include priority-setting for system change (including taxation and regulation in the interest of public health) as well as a priority agenda for the urgent focus for implementation work in areas such as health service delivery, local area change and individual behavioural change.

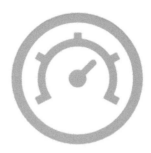

2. RECOMMENDATIONS FOR CAPACITY BUILDING

Ensuring the capacity of social scientists with expertise in health (including public health, population behaviour change, more targeted behavioural change, and health systems delivery) is critical. A key element is ensuring that there is a suitably trained workforce which not only has traditional health research skills, but also social science and data and analysis skills too.

Recommendation 2.1

We recommend that the UK strategic coordinating body should review the existing skills and expertise available for research into behavioural and social science in relation to health. This review should assess how the necessary skills and expertise can be developed, including the need for more diverse and appropriate training pathways, and include training in how to engage effectively with potential users of research, as well as how medical researchers and practitioners (including Directors of Public Health, service commissioners, and managers) could engage more strategically with social science expertise.

The importance of professional behaviour is recognised in the education strategies of Health Education England (HEE), which 'exists for one reason only: to support the delivery of excellent healthcare and health improvement to the patients and public of England by ensuring that the workforce of today and tomorrow has the right numbers, skills, values and behaviours, at the right time and in the right place'.[159] 'Making Every Contact Count' and 'Health Promoting Health Service' are NHS programmes to increase the skills of NHS staff in using every opportunity to prompt health-related behaviour change, emphasising the need for all staff to have some behaviour change skills.[160]

The ability to integrate the knowledge and skill of behavioural and social sciences with those of the clinical sciences has been an integral part of General Medical Council (GMC) recommendations for medical education since the mid-twentieth century,[161] and is now agreed to be part of the core curriculum[162] with many textbooks now incorporated into undergraduate and other training.[163] The Scottish Government Health and Social Care Directorate has commissioned the development of the Health Behaviour Change Competency Framework[164] for use in assessing the knowledge and skills required, and for designing training.[165]

Recommendation 2.2

But we suspect that a further issue is not just how to raise the knowledge of all members of the NHS workforce but how to create a cadre of professionals and practitioners who will be strategic drivers of innovation and change. **We recommend that the UK strategic coordinating body should consider how best to encourage and incentivise those involved in promoting health and commissioning delivering healthcare services to make appropriate use of research findings and expertise, including social science evidence.** In doing so, it should make use of behavioural and social science research about incentivisation and research translation. Together, these add up to a recommendation that the UK adopts a more strategic approach to build human capacity related to social sciences and health. There is already much excellent work going on, with funders such as the MRC, Wellcome Trust and the Health Foundation funding fellowships, post-docs, and so on. Routinely attaching funds to centres would be a step forward. We recommend that some of these must be explicitly aimed at increasing the number of social scientists working in this area, from master's degrees upwards. This should include explicitly multi-disciplinary programmes aimed at enhancing skills within disciplines (such as psychology, sociology, political science, economics, demography and anthropology), as well as bringing different social sciences together.

It should also include a focus on programmes to enhance methodological skills, with an appreciation of the range of methods (not just randomised trials but other experimental methods, such as the use of observational and qualitative methods) allied to substantive fields of work. The latter is particularly important in an area where randomised controlled trials (RCTs) can be only one part of the mix. The social science and medical literature is rich in examples of why RCTs are only a part of the mix, particularly in the case of complex interventions, which cannot be 'blind' to those working on them or the populations they are aimed at. Sophisticated statistical studies of various types would be needed, as well as qualitative studies. This will require engagement with relevant funding bodies, other strategic social science bodies and universities. This goes beyond recommendation 4 in the Academy of Medical Sciences' report.[166] We believe that it will be important for the new strategic body to work with others to ensure funding incentives to build capacity especially in the social sciences, and for the social sciences to engage actively with these initiatives. The Academy of Social Sciences is ready to play its part.

Recommendation 2.3

We recommend that the strategy for capacity building should include developing greater numbers of people who can ally high-level data and informatics skills with substantive knowledge of health research. This will require a strategic priority among research funders and a focus on training pathways to provide new capacity, and include consideration of how to draw in mathematics, physics and data analytic specialists into social and behavioural health and health delivery research.

Recommendation 2.4

We suspect that work both on organisational change within NHS organisations and on aspects of population change, allied with greater data (from NHS service provision, administrative data and other sources) present an opportunity for a new research agenda on the importance of social relationships (including the roles of changing social norms and social support) in individual behaviour and behavioural change. Many of our case studies have showed the importance not only of individual incentives but the importance of social relationships and norms for behaviour. Taking this seriously as a resource for change could be akin to the change wrought by behavioural economics, bringing psychology into economics premised on individual rational actors. **We recommend that research funders consider a new interdisciplinary research agenda on the importance of macro- and micro-environments and of social relationships (including the roles of changing social norms and social support) in bringing about behaviour change.**

3. RECOMMENDATIONS FOR DATA PROVISION AND ACCESS

To support these programmes of work, we have argued that further developments in the better provision of and access to data will be essential.

Recommendation 3.1

We support the calls of the Wachter review for the development of efficient and effective systems for collecting, generating and accessing data relevant to behaviour change in healthcare and public health. The use of such data (usually in the form of de-personalised data sets, where individuals are not identifiable) is essential for public-benefit research to improve the health of the nation.

But even with better digital data, access to data remains a problem. Current proposals for legislation to bring clarity to efforts to promote wider sharing of de-identified or anonymised data for public-benefit research may help.[167]

It is imperative and urgent that efforts continue to ensure that data are available from NHS Digital (formerly the Health and Social Care Information Centre) that can be linked with the social, economic and geographic anonymised data from central and local government to explore the social bases of health. This will require cultural and behavioural change on the part of central Government and by NHS Digital itself to open up data to more widespread use by social scientists and others doing public health research. Of course this must always involve serious safeguards, including the data matching process, data security, lay involvement in assessing public benefit, and so on, which we have outlined as comprising the 'social consent' model. It will require further, better and deeper engagement with the public about the benefits and risks of this type of research, and a culture of transparency (the Administrative Data Research Network provides a useful model, as does the Wellcome Initiative on Understanding Public Health).[168] But currently delays means it can take years to gain access to data even with the highest safeguards and security built in.

Recommendation 3.2

The UK strategic coordinating body should play an active role in unlocking the current difficulties in accessing health data and linking them to social data to provide research access that is both necessary to improve population health and consistent with public acceptance of public-benefit research carried out with appropriate safeguards.

Recommendation 3.3

We also call for a greater level of urgency in the deliberations of NHS Digital and the Department of Health over health data linkage and for the 'social consent' model we propose in this report to form an important foundation for these policy discussions.

We recognise that this will require wider debate to unlock the current difficulties in linking health and social data.[169] The Government response to the Caldicott Review will be important but is unlikely to recommend the access that we believe is necessary, and is consistent with public acceptance of public-benefit research carried out with high safeguards. Into this vacuum we may see more local area deals with private providers (such as the arrangement between the Royal Free group and Google DeepMind). Such arrangements have benefits if they are carried out transparently and, of course, with the practical knowledge and skills in digital technologies they bring. But there are broader needs that require opening up national and regional data to address the broader social agenda that we believe is necessary.

Recommendation 3.4

We recommend that parliamentarians, policy-makers, health organisations and the broader public should be engaged in an urgent debate about the benefits of opening up access to link 'de-personalised' health data with broader social data to improve health policy, practice and behaviour. Social scientists should be active participants in these discussions about data linkage, as they have useful research and evidence about public views on these matters.

Taken together, the Campaign for Social Science believes that these recommendations would help improve not only the research evidence available but also the way that research can be used to drive changes in health services, public policy and the health-related behaviours – all for the sake of the health of people.

APPENDIX A: CONTRIBUTORS

Job titles and affiliations are those at the time of engagement with the project.

PARTICIPANTS AT ROUNDTABLE DISCUSSIONS

Health service delivery

Stephen Anderson, Executive Director, Campaign for Social Science; **Eric Barratt**, NHS Healthy Workforce Programme Manager, NHS England; **Anda Bayliss**, Research and Innovation Manager – Evidence, Royal College of Nursing; **Siôn Charles**, Deputy Director, Bevan Commission; **Ed Day**, Senior Clinical Lecturer in Addiction Psychiatry, National Addiction Centre, Institute of Psychiatry, and Consultant at Birmingham & Solihull Mental Health NHS Foundation Trust; **Erik Ducker**, Portfolio Developer – Communities and Knowledge, Wellcome Trust; **Posy Goraya**, Senior Manager, NHS RightCare, NHS England; **Sir Malcolm Grant** CBE FAcSS, Chair, NHS England; **Laura Harper**, Research Manager, Health Foundation; **Paula Lorgelly**, Deputy Director, Office of Health Economics; **Christine McGuire**, Science Research and Evidence Directorate, Department of Health; **Amie McWilliam-Reynolds**, Head of Research, Healthwatch; **Susan Michie** FAcSS, Director, Centre for Behaviour Change, University College London, and Chair of The Health of People project; **Al Mulley**, Managing Director, The Dartmouth Center for Health Care Delivery; **Carol Propper** CBE, Associate Dean of Faculty and Research and Chair in Economics, Imperial College Business School; **João Rangel de Almeida**, Portfolio Development Manager, Wellcome Trust; **Chris Walters**, Chief Economist, NHS Improvement; **Tim Whitaker** FAcSS, Director of Communications, Hanover Housing, and member of The Health of People Working Group; **Sharon Witherspoon** MBE FAcSS, Head of Policy, Campaign for Social Science.

Prevention

Louise Ansari, Director of Communications, Centre for Ageing Better; **Mark Baker**, Director of the Centre for Guidelines, NICE; **Amanda Bunten**, Behavioural Insights Team, Public Health England; **Tim Chadborn**, Behavioural Insights Lead Researcher, Public Health England; **Ed Day**, Senior Clinical Lecturer in Addiction Psychiatry, King's College London, and Consultant at Birmingham & Solihull Mental Health NHS Foundation Trust; **Erik Ducker**, Portfolio Developer – Communities and Knowledge, Wellcome Trust; **Kevin Fenton**, Director of Health and Wellbeing, Public Health England; **Paul Lincoln**, Chief Executive, UK Health Forum; **Christine McGuire**, Science Research and Evidence Directorate, Department of Health; **Wendy Meredith**, Director of Population Health Transformation, Greater Manchester; **Susan Michie** FAcSS, Director of the Centre for Behaviour Change, University College London, and Chair of The Health of People project; **Laurence Moore** FAcSS, Director of the MRC/ CSO Social & Public Health Sciences Unit, University of Glasgow; **João Rangel de Almeida**, Portfolio Development Manager, Wellcome Trust; **Helen Walters**, Public Health Consultant Advisor, NIHR – NETSCC; **Robert West**, Director of Tobacco Studies, the Cancer Research UK Health Behaviour Research Centre, UCL, and member of The Health of People Working Group; **Sharon Witherspoon** MBE FAcSS, Head of Policy, Campaign for Social Science; **Dagmar Zeuner**, Director of Public Health, London Borough of Merton, and member of The Health of People Working Group.

Use of health data

Jo Churchill, Member of Parliament for Bury St Edmunds; **Tommy Denning**, Information Governance Policy Manager, Department of Health; **Erik Ducker**, Portfolio Developer – Communities and Knowledge, Wellcome Trust; **Katie Farrington**, Director of Digital and Data Policy, Department of Health; **Harry Hemingway**, Director of the Farr Institute of Health Informatics, UCL; **Susan Michie** FAcSS, Director, Centre for Behaviour Change, University College London, and Chair of The Health of People project; **Ronan Lyons**, Professor of Public Health, Swansea University and Director, CIPHER, and Co-Director of the SAIL Databank; **Freda Mold**, Lecturer in Integrated Care, University of Surrey; **Louise Park**, Associate Director (Health), Ipsos MORI; **Nicola Perrin**, Head of Policy, Wellcome Trust; **Andrew Roddam**, Vice President & Global Head Epidemiology, GSK; **Shobna Vasishta**, Programme Manager, SHARE; **Robert West**, Director of Tobacco Studies, Cancer Research UK Health Behaviour Research Centre, UCL, and member of The Health of People Working Group; **Sharon Witherspoon** MBE FAcSS, Head of Policy, Campaign for Social Science.

Respondents to Call for Evidence

Carol Atkinson, Associate Dean: Research, Manchester Metropolitan University Business School; **Clare Bambra** FAcSS, Professor of Public Health Geography, Durham University; **Julie Barnett**, Professor of Health Psychology, University of Bath; **Bernadette Bartlam**, Lecturer in Health Services Research, Keele University; **Yehuda Baruch** FAcSS, Professor of Management, Director of Research, Southampton Business School, University of Southampton; **Nicola Bolton**, Principal Lecturer, Cardiff School of Sport, Cardiff Metropolitan University; **Mark Brosnan**, Reader in Psychology and the Director of Research for Psychology, University of Bath; **Daniela Carl** Deputy Chief Executive, Regional Studies Association; **Ruby C M Chau**, Visiting Scholar, The University of Sheffield; **Sarah Chaytor**, Head of Public Policy, Office of the Vice-Provost, UCL; **Linda Clare** FAcSS, Professor of Clinical Psychology of Ageing and Dementia, University of Exeter; **Jessie Cooper**, Lecturer in the Sociology of Public Health, Institute of Psychology, Health and Society, The University of Liverpool; **Rob Davies**, Public Affairs Manager, CLOSER UCL Institute of Education; **Zowie Davy**, Senior Lecturer, School of Health and Social Care, University of Lincoln; **Claire Donovan**, Reader, Institute of Environment, Health and Societies, Brunel University; **Danny Dorling** FAcSS, Halford Mackinder Professor of Geography of the School of Geography and the Environment, University of Oxford; **Simon Dyson**, Professor of Applied Sociology, De Montfort University; **Chris Eccleston**, Professor, Department for Health University of Bath; the **Economic and Social Research Council**; **Natalie Forster**, PhD Candidate in Sociology, University of Edinburgh; **Stewart Fotheringham** FAcSS, Professor of Computational Spatial Science in the School of Geographical Sciences and Urban Planning, Arizona State University; **Simone Fullagar**, Professor of Sport and Physical Cultural Studies, University of Bath; **Sarah Galvani**, Professor of Adult Social Care, Manchester Metropolitan University; **Kenneth Gilhooly** FAcSS, Research Professor in Quantitative Gerontology, Brunel University; **Anna Gilmore**, Professor, Department for Health, University of Bath; **Trisha Greenhalgh**, Professor of Primary Care Health Sciences, University of Oxford; **Lea Hagoel**, Department of Community Medicine and Epidemiology, Technion; **Catherine Hamilton-Giachritsis**, Senior Lecturer in Forensic Psychology, University of Birmingham; **Linda Hantrais** FAcSS, Emeritus Professor of European Social Policy, Loughborough University; **Steve Hanney**, Emeritus Professor, Brunel University; **Alex Haslam** FAcSS, The University of Queensland; **Jenny Hatchard**, Research Fellow, Department for Health, University of Bath; **Jonathan Hill**, Senior Lecturer in Physiotherapy, Keele University; **Clare Jinks**, Reader in Applied Health Research, Keele University; **Sarah Macdonald**,

Research Fellow, Nottingham University; **Linda Machin**, Honorary Research Fellow, Keele University; **Daryl Martin**, Lecturer in Sociology, University of York; **Tony McEnery** FAcSS, Director of the ESRC Centre for Corpus Approaches to Social Science and Distinguished Professor of English Language and Linguistics, Lancaster University; **Jane Meyrick**, Senior Lecturer, Department of Psychology, University of the West of England; **Jennifer Newton**, Head of School of Social Sciences, Faculty of Social Sciences and Humanities, London Metropolitan University; **Josephine Ocloo**, Research Fellow (Improvement Science), London Imperial College; **Rachel O'Hara**, Senior Lecturer in Public Health, University of Bath; **Lois Orton**, Senior Research Fellow, University of Liverpool; **Eugenia I Pearson**; **Cassandra Phoenix**, Reader, Department for Health, University of Bath; **Victoria Pinoncely** Research Officer, Royal Town Planning Institute; **Subhash Pokhrel**, Senior Lecturer, Brunel University; **Shirin M Rai** FAcSS, Professor, Department of Politics and International Studies, University of Warwick; **Emma Rich**, Senior Lecturer, Department for Health, University of Bath; **Carol Rivas**, Senior Research Fellow, University of Southampton; **Peter Rouse**, Medlock Research Associate, University of Bath; **Paul Salkovskis**, Professor of Clinical Psychology & Applied Science, University of Bath; **Ted Schrecker**, Professor of Global Health Policy, School of Medicine, Pharmacy and Health, Durham University; **Rebecca Shortt**, Senior Policy Manager, The Brain Tumour Charity; **Martyn Standage**, Professor, Department for Health, University of Bath; **Afroditi Stathi**, Senior Lecturer, Department for Health, University of Bath; **Bas Verplanken**, Head of Department of Psychology, University of Bath; **Justin Waring** FAcSS, Associate Dean (Engagement), Director of Centre for Health Innovation, Nottingham University Business School; **Kelly J Watson**, PhD and Research Associate, School of Environment, Education & Development, University of Manchester; **Vishanth Weerakkody**, Professor of Digital Governance, Director of Business Life, Brunel University; **Judith Wester**, Director, CEDAR Education CIC; **Andrew Weyman**, Senior Lecturer, Department of Psychology, University of Bath; **Wendy Wills**, Professor of Food and Public Health and Director of the Centre for Research in Primary and Community Care, University of Hertfordshire; **Kerry Woolfall**, Research Fellow Institute of Psychology, Health and Society, University of Liverpool; **Penny Wright**, Associate Professor in Psychosocial Cancer Care, University of Bath; **Jennifer Yiallouros**, Senior Health Evaluation and Research Analyst, Cancer Research UK; **Keming Yu**, Research Director (Impact) Reader in Statistics, Brunel University; and **Sam W K Yu**, Associate Professor, Department of Social Work, Hong Kong Baptist University.

REFERENCES

1 National Institutes of Health: Office of Behavioral and Social Science Research, 'BSSR definition', https://obssr.od.nih.gov/about-us/bssr-definition/

2 Academy of Medical Sciences, *Improving the Health of the Public by 2040*, 2016, https://acmedsci.ac.uk/file-download/41399-5807581429f81.pdf

3 See recommendations in Academy of Medical Sciences, *Improving the Health of the Public by 2040*, 2016.

4 Ibid.

5 Wachter, Robert, *Making IT Work: Harnessing the power of health information technology to improve care in England*, 2016,www.gov.uk/government/uploads/system/uploads/attachment_data/file/550866/Wachter_Review_Accessible.pdf

6 Macintyre, Sally, 'Keeping social sciences in the MRC family', 2013, www.insight.mrc.ac.uk/2013/09/24/keeping-social-sciences-in-the-mrc-family/

7 HM Government, *A Smokefree Future: A comprehensive tobacco control strategy for England*, 2010, http://webarchive.nationalarchives.gov.uk/20100509080731/www.dh.gov.uk/prod_consum_dh/groups/dh_digitalassets/@dh/@en/@ps/documents/digitalasset/dh_111789.pdf

8 Davies, Karen, *et al.*, *Mirror, Mirror on the Wall: How the performance of the U.S. healthcare system compares internationally*, The Commonwealth Fund, 2014, www.commonwealthfund.org/~/media/files/publications/fund-report/2014/jun/1755_davis_mirror_mirror_2014.pdf

9 See Office for National Statistics, 'Expenditure on healthcare in the UK: 2013 – Total healthcare expenditure per person', 2015, www.ons.gov.uk/peoplepopulationandcommunity/healthandsocialcare/healthcaresystem/articles/expenditureonhealthcareintheuk/2015-03-26#total-healthcare-expenditure-per-person. Also see three articles by the King's Fund: 'NHS spending: squeezed as never before', 2015, www.kingsfund.org.uk/blog/2015/10/nhs-spending-squeezed-never; 'How does this year's NHS budget compare historically?', 2016, www.kingsfund.org.uk/blog/2016/05/how-does-this-years-nhs-budget-compare-historically; 'UK spending on healthcare and social care', 2016, www.kingsfund.org.uk/blog/2016/06/uk-spending-health-care-and-social-care; and an analytical paper by the Office for Budget Responsibility, 'Fiscal sustainability and public spending on health', 2016, http://budgetresponsibility.org.uk/docs/dlm_uploads/Health-FSAP.pdf

10 Pickett, Kate, and Wilkinson, Richard, *The Spirit Level: Why equality is better for everyone*, Allen Lane, 2009; Kelly, Michael P., et al., *The Social Determinants of Health: Developing an evidence base for political action, final report to the World Health Organization Commission on the Social Determinants of Health*, Measurement and Evidence Knowledge Network, 2007, www.who.int/social_determinants/resources/mekn_report_10oct07.pdf

11 Marmot, Michael, *Fair Society, Healthy Lives* (The Marmot Review), 2010, www.instituteofhealthequity.org/projects/fair-society-healthy-lives-the-marmot-review

12 NICE, 'Health inequalities and population health', Local government briefing [LGB4], 2012, www.nice.org.uk/advice/lgb4/chapter/introduction; Doohan, Morgan A., and Kelly, Michael P., 'The social determinants of health', in Merson, Michael H., Black, Robert E., and Mills, Anne J. (eds), *Global Health: Diseases, programs, systems and policies*, 3rd edition, Jones & Bartlett, 2012, pp. 75–113.

13 Office for National Statistics, 'Estimates of the very old (including centenarians), UK: 2002 to 2015', 2016, www.ons.gov.uk/peoplepopulationandcommunity/birthsdeathsandmarriages/ageing/bulletins/estimatesoftheveryoldincludingcentenarians/2002to2015#statisticians-quote

14 Public Health England, 'UK and Ireland prevalence and trends', 2016, www.noo.org.uk/NOO_about_obesity/adult_obesity/UK_prevalence_and_trends

15 Department of Health, *Long Term Conditions Compendium of Information: Third edition*, 2012, www.gov.uk/government/uploads/system/uploads/attachment_data/file/216528/dh_134486.pdf

16 NHS England, *Five Year Forward View*, 2014, p. 3, www.england.nhs.uk/wp-content/uploads/2014/10/5yfv-web.pdf

17 Alwan, Ali, *Global Status Report on Noncommunicable Diseases 2010*, World Health Organization, 2011; Parkin, D.M., et al., 'The fraction of cancer attributable to lifestyle and environmental factors in the UK in 2010', *British Journal of Cancer*, 2011, 105: Si–S81; Cancer Research UK, 'Cigarettes, diet, alcohol and obesity behind more than 100,000 cancers', 2011, www.cancerresearchuk.org/about-us/cancer-news/press-release/2011-12-07-cigarettes-diet-alcohol-and-obesity-behind-more-than-100000-cancers?rss=true; Lim, S.S., et al., 'A comparative risk assessment of burden of disease and injury attributable to 67 risk factors and risk factor clusters in 21 regions, 1990–2010: A systematic analysis for the Global Burden of Disease Study 2010', *The Lancet*, 2012, 380: 2224–2260.

18 Office for Budget Responsibility, 'Fiscal sustainability and public spending on health', 2016, http://budgetresponsibility.org.uk/docs/dlm_uploads/Health-FSAP.pdf

19 Kelly, Michael P., and Barker, Mary, 'Why is changing health related behaviour so difficult?', *Public Health*, 2016, 136: 109–116, www.sciencedirect.com/science/article/pii/S0033350616300178

20 Academy of Medical Sciences, *Health of the Public in 2040*, 2016, www.acmedsci.ac.uk/policy/policy-projects/health-of-the-public-in-2040/; All Party Parliamentary

Group on Primary Care and Public Health, *Inquiry Report into NHS England's 'Five Year Forward View': Behaviour change, information and signposting*, 2016, www.pagb.co.uk/content/uploads/2016/06/5YFV_Behaviour_Change_Info_Signposting_15March16.pdf; NHS England, *Five Year Forward View*, 2014, p. 3, www.england.nhs.uk/wp-content/uploads/2014/10/5yfv-web.pdf; National Institute for Health and Clinical Excellence, 'Behaviour change', Local government briefing, 2013, www.nice.org.uk/advice/lgb7/chapter/Introduction; Public Health England, 'Our support for popula-tion behaviour change', 2016, https://publichealthmatters.blog.gov.uk/2016/09/02/our-support-for-population-behaviour-change/; National Institute for Health and Clinical Excellence, 'Behaviour change at population, community and individual levels', 2007, www.ncsct.co.uk/usr/pub/guidance-on-behaviour-change-at-population.pdf

21 Fenton, Kevin, 'Our support for population behaviour change', Public Health England, 2016, https://publichealthmatters.blog.gov.uk/2016/09/02/our-support-for-population-behaviour-change/

22 Nesta, *Introducing…Health Lab*, 2016, www.nesta.org.uk/sites/default/files/introducing_health_lab_v3.pdf

23 Hallsworth, Michael, *et al.*, *Applying Behavioral Insights: Simple ways to improve health outcomes*, World Innovation Summit for Health, 2016, www.behaviouralinsights.co.uk/publications/applying-behavioural-insights-simple-ways-to-improve-health-outcomes/

24 The Academy of Medical Sciences, *Improving the Health of the Public by 2040*, 2016, https://acmedsci.ac.uk/file-download/41399-5807581429f81.pdf

25 International Collaboration for Participatory Health Research (ICPHR), *Position Paper 1: What is participatory health research?* Version: May 2013, International Collaboration for Participatory Health Research.

26 NHS England, *Five Year Forward View*, 2014, p. 3, www.england.nhs.uk/wp-content/uploads/2014/10/5yfv-web.pdf

27 NHS England, 'Simon Stevens call for bold action to make NHS fit for the future', 2015, www.england.nhs.uk/2015/05/fit-for-future/

28 Cabinet Office, *Government Response to the Science and Technology Select Committee Report on Behaviour Change*, 2011, www.gov.uk/government/uploads/system/uploads/attachment_data/file/60538/Government-Response-House-of-Lords-Inquiry-Behaviour-Change.pdf

29 Academy of Medical Sciences, *Health of the Public in 2040*, 2016, pp. 17–18, www.acmedsci.ac.uk/policy/policy-projects/health-of-the-public-in-2040/

30 National Institutes of Health, 'Estimates of funding for various research, condition, and disease categories (RCDC)', 2016, https://report.nih.gov/categorical_spending.aspx

31 Hine, Deidre, *The 2009 Influenza Pandemic: An independent review of the UK response to the 2009 influenza pandemic*, 2010, www.gov.uk/government/publications/independent-review-into-the-response-to-the-2009-swine-flu-pandemic

32 National Institute for Health and Clinical Excellence, *Behaviour Change at Population, Community and Individual Levels*, 2007, www.ncsct.co.uk/usr/pub/guidance-on-behaviour-change-at-population.pdf

33 Aveyard, Paul, *et al.*, 'Screening and brief intervention for obesity in primary care: A parallel, two-arm, randomised trial', *The Lancet*, 2016, Nov 19, 388(10059): 2492–2500, www.thelancet.com/journals/lancet/article/PIIS0140–6736(16)31893–1/fulltext; Jolly, Kate, *et al.*, 'A randomised controlled trial to compare a range of commercial or primary care led weight reduction programmes with a minimal intervention control for weight loss in obesity: The Lighten Up trial', *BMC Public Health*, 2010, July 27, 10: 439; Jebb, Susan A., 'Primary care referral to a commercial provider for weight loss treatment versus standard care: A randomised controlled trial', *The Lancet*, 2011, Oct 22, 378(9801): 1485–1492, www.thelancet.com/journals/lancet/article/PIIS0140-6736(11)61344-5/abstract

34 Teenage Pregnancy Independent Advisory Group, *Final Report: Teenage Pregnancy: Past successes – future challenges*, 2010, www.gov.uk/government/uploads/system/uploads/attachment_data/file/181078/TPIAG-FINAL-REPORT.pdf

35 Wellings, K., *et al.*, 'Changes in conceptions in women younger than 18 years and the circumstances of young mothers in England in 2000–12: An observational study', *The Lancet*, 2016, 388(10044): 586–595; Social Exclusion Unit, 'Teenage pregnancy', 1999, http://dera.ioe.ac.uk/15086/; http://dx.doi.org/10.1016/S0140-6736(16)30449-4

36 Skinner, Rachel, *et al.*, 'England's teenage pregnancy strategy: A hard-won success', *The Lancet*, 2016, 388(10044): 538–540, http://dx.doi.org/10.1016/S0140-6736(16)30589-X

37 UCL News, 'Teenage pregnancies hit record low, reflecting efforts of England's strategy to reduce under-18 conceptions', 2016, www.ucl.ac.uk/news/news-articles/0516/230515_teenage_pregnancies

38 UNICEF, 'Child well-being in rich countries: A comparative overview', *Innocenti Report Card*, 11, 2013, www.unicef-irc.org/publications/pdf/rc11_eng.pdf

39 Public Health England, *NHS Health Checks: Applying all our health (guidance)*, 2015, www.gov.uk/government/publications/nhs-health-checks-applying-all-our-health/nhs-health-checks-applying-all-our-health

40 Baker, Colin, *et al.*, 'A process evaluation of the NHS Health Check care pathway in a primary care setting', *Journal of Public Health*, 2015, 37(2): 202–209, https://academic.oup.com/jpubhealth/article-lookup/doi/10.1093/pubmed/fdv053; Kypridemos, Chris, 'Cardiovascular screening to reduce the burden from cardiovascular disease: Microsimulation study to quantify policy options', *BMJ*, 2016, 353, www.bmj.com/content/353/bmj.i2793

41 Thaler, Richard, *et al.*, *Nudge: Improving decisions about health, wealth and happiness*, Yale University Press, 2008; Kahneman, Daniel, *Thinking, Fast and Slow*, Farrar, Straus and Giroux, 2011.

42 Nuffield Council of Bioethics, *Public Health: Ethical issues*, 2007, http://nuffieldbioethics.org/wp-content/uploads/2014/07/Public-health-ethical-issues.pdf

43 Ibid., p. 42.

44 McGill, Rory, *et al.*, 'Are interventions to promote healthy eating equally effective for all? Systematic review of socioeconomic inequalities in impact', *BMC Public Health*, 2015, 15: 457, http://bmcpublichealth.biomedcentral.com/articles/10.1186/s12889-015-1781-7;

Olstad, Dana L., et al., 'Can policy ameliorate socioeconomic inequities in obesity and obesity-related behaviours? A systematic review of the impact of universal policies on adults and children, *Obesity Reviews*, 2016, 17(12), http://onlinelibrary.wiley.com/doi/10.1111/obr.12457/full#references; Adams, Jean, et al., 'Why are some population interventions for diet and obesity more equitable and effective than others? The role of individual agency', *PLoS One*, 2016, http://dx.doi.org/10.1371/journal.pmed.1001990; Marteau, Theresa M., Hollands, Gareth J., and Fletcher, Paul C., 'Changing human behavior to prevent disease: The importance of targeting automatic processes', *Science*, 2012, Sept 21, 337(6101): 1492–1495, http://science.sciencemag.org/content/337/6101/1492.full

45 House of Lords Science and Technology Committee, *Behaviour Change, Second Report of Session 2010–12*, www.publications.parliament.uk/pa/ld201012/ldselect/ldsctech/179/179.pdf

46 Institute for Fiscal Studies, *Tax and Benefit Policy: Insights from behavioural economics*, 2012, www.ifs.org.uk/comms/comm125.pdf

47 House of Lords Science and Technology Committee, *Behaviour Change, Second Report of Session 2010–12*, www.publications.parliament.uk/pa/ld201012/ldselect/ldsctech/179/179.pdf

48 Public Health England, *The Public Health Burden of Alcohol and the Effectiveness and Cost-Effectiveness of Alcohol Control Policies: An evidence review*, 2016, www.gov.uk/government/uploads/system/uploads/attachment_data/file/574427/Alcohol_public_health_burden_evidence_review.pdf

49 www.shef.ac.uk/scharr/sections/ph/research/alpol/research/completed/iarp

50 Bader, Pearl, Boisclair, David, and Ferrence, Roberta, 'Effects of tobacco taxation and pricing on smoking behavior in high risk populations: A knowledge synthesis', *International Journal of Environmental Research and Public Health*, 2011, Nov, 8(11): 4118–4139, www.ncbi.nlm.nih.gov/pmc/articles/PMC3228562/; Goodchild, Mark, Perucica, Anne-Marie, and Nargisb, Nigar, 'Modelling the impact of raising tobacco taxes on public health and finance', *Bulletin of the World Health Organization*, 2016, 94: 250–257.

51 Action on Smoking and Health, *Smoking Still Kills: Protecting children, reducing inequalities*, 2015, http://ash.org.uk/information-and-resources/reports-submissions/reports/smoking-still-kills/

52 Kate Frazer, et al., 'Legislative smoking bans for reducing harms from secondhand smoke exposure, smoking prevalence and tobacco consumption', *The Cochrane Library*, 2016, 4 February, 2:CD005992, http://onlinelibrary.wiley.com/doi/10.1002/14651858.CD005992.pub3/abstract

53 Kotz, Daniel, et al., 'How cost-effective is 'No Smoking Day'?' *Tobacco Control*, 2011, 20: 302–304, http://tobaccocontrol.bmj.com/content/20/4/302; Brown, Jamie, et al., 'How effective and cost-effective was the national mass media smoking cessation campaign 'Stoptober'?', *Drug and Alcohol Dependence*, 2014, 135: 52–58, www.drugandalcohol dependence.com/article/S0376-8716(13)00470-5/fulltext

54 West, Robert, 'Performance of English stop smoking services in first 10 years: Analysis of service monitoring data', *BMJ*, 2013, Aug 19, 347: f4921, www.bmj.com/content/347/bmj.f4921

55 Stead, Lindsay F., *et al.*, 'Physician advice for smoking cessation', *The Cochrane Database of Systematic Reviews*, 2013, http://onlinelibrary.wiley.com/doi/10.1002/14651858.CD000165.pub4/abstract

56 NICE, 'Smoking: Brief interventions and referrals', *Public Health Guideline* [PH1], 2006, www.nice.org.uk/guidance/ph1

57 Ibid.

58 Aveyard, Paul, *et al.*, 'Brief opportunistic smoking cessation interventions: A systematic review and meta-analysis to compare advice to quit and offer of assistance', *Addiction*, 2012, June, 107(6): 1066–1073.

59 Brown, Jamie, 'Comparison of brief interventions in primary care on smoking and excessive alcohol consumption: A population survey in England', *British Journal of General Practice*, 2016, 66(642): e1–e9, http://bjgp.org/content/66/642/e1

60 Coleman, Tim, *et al.*, 'Impact of contractual financial incentives on the ascertainment and management of smoking in primary care', *Addiction*, 2007, 102(5): 803–808, http://onlinelibrary.wiley.com/doi/10.1111/j.1360-0443.2007.01766.x/abstract

61 Kelly, Mike P., *et al.*, 'A conceptual framework for public health: NICE's emerging approach', *Public Health*, 2009, 123: e14–e20, www.publichealthjrnl.com/article/S0033-3506(08)00279-5/abstract; Baxter, Susan, *et al.*, 'Synthesizing diverse evidence: The use of primary qualitative data analysis methods and logic models in public health reviews', *Public Health*, 2010, 124(2): 99–106, www.publichealthjrnl.com/article/S0033-3506(10)00004-1/fulltext

62 Medical Research Council, *Developing and Evaluating Complex Interventions: New guidance*, 2006, www.mrc.ac.uk/documents/pdf/complex-interventions-guidance/. See also the Cochrane Effective Practice and Organisation of Care reviews: http://epoc.cochrane.org/our-reviews

63 Nilson, Per, 'Making sense of implementation: Theories, models and frameworks', *Implementation Science*, 2015, 10(53), https://implementationscience.biomedcentral.com/articles/10.1186/s13012-015-0242-0; Michie, Susan, *et al.*, 'The behaviour change wheel: A new method for characterising and designing behaviour change interventions', *Implementation Science*, 2011, 6(42), https://implementationscience.biomedcentral.com/articles/10.1186/1748-5908-6-42

64 Michie, Susan, *et al.*, 'The behaviour change wheel: A new method for characterising and designing behaviour change interventions', *Implementation Science*, 2011, 6(42), https://implementationscience.biomedcentral.com/articles/10.1186/1748-5908-6-42

65 Ibid.; Michie, Susan, *The Behaviour Change Wheel: A guide to designing interventions*, Silverback Publishing, 2014, www.behaviourchangewheel.com

66 Hallsworth, Michael, *et al.*, *Applying Behavioral Insights: Simple ways to improve health outcomes*, World Innovation Summit for Health, 2016, www.behaviouralinsights.co.uk/publications/

applying-behavioural-insights-simple-ways-to-improve-health-outcomes; Burd, Hannah, and Hallsworth, Michael, *Supporting Self-management: A guide to enabling behaviour change for health and wellbeing using person- and community-centred approaches*, Realising the Value, Nesta, 2016, www.nesta.org.uk/sites/default/files/rtv-supporting-self-management.pdf

67 International Collaboration for Participatory Health Research (ICPHR), *Position Paper 1: What is participatory health research?* Version: May 2013. Berlin: International Collaboration for Participatory Health Research, www.icphr.org/uploads/2/0/3/9/20399575/ichpr_position_paper_1_definition_-_version_may_2013.pdf

68 www.england.nhs.uk/ourwork/innovation/healthy-new-towns/

69 Government Office for Science, *Tackling Obesities: Future choices – project report, 2nd edition,* 2007, www.gov.uk/government/publications/reducing-obesity-future-choices

70 Falbe, Jennifer, *et al.*, 'Impact of the Berkeley Excise Tax on sugar-sweetened beverage consumption', *American Journal of Public Health,* 2016, 106(10), https://nature.berkeley.edu/garbelottoat/wp-content/uploads/falbe-etal-2016.pdf; Colchero, Arantxa, *et al.*, 'Beverage purchases from stores in Mexico under the excise tax on sugar sweetened beverages: Observational study', *BMJ,* 2016, 352, www.bmj.com/content/352/bmj.h6704

71 See, for example, the Cancer Research UK campaign, *Be Clear on Cancer,* www.cancerresearchuk.org/health-professional/early-diagnosis-activities/be-clear-on-cancer; and the NHS campaigns *Stoptober,* www.nhs.uk/oneyou/stoptober/home#fgEyILmUfD2tpTef.97; and *Stay Well This Winter,* www.nhs.uk/staywell/#jGdjHmhgEpbeZreO.97

72 Examples include the National Institute for Health Research, 'A systematic review, evidence synthesis and meta-analysis of quantitative and qualitative studies evaluating the clinical effectiveness, the cost effectiveness, safety and acceptability of interventions to prevent postnatal depression', *Health Technology Assessment,* 2016, 20(37), www.journalslibrary.nihr.ac.uk/hta/volume-20/issue-37; and O'Mara-Eves, Alison, *et al.*, 'The effectiveness of community engagement in public health interventions for disadvantaged groups: A meta-analysis', *BMC Public Health,* 2015, 15(129), http://bmcpublichealth.biomedcentral.com/articles/10.1186/s12889-015-1352-y

73 Jakicic, John, *et al.*, 'Effect of wearable technology combined with a lifestyle intervention on long-term weight loss: The IDEA randomized clinical trial', *JAMA,* 2016, 316(11): 1161–1171, http://jamanetwork.com/journals/jama/article-abstract/2553448

74 Tremblay, Mark S., *et al.*, 'Global Matrix 2.0: Report card grades on the physical activity of children and youth comparing 38 countries', *Journal of Physical Activity and Health,* 2016, 13(Suppl 2): S343–S366, http://ki.se/sites/default/files/b_global_matrix_article.pdf

75 House of Commons Health Committee, *Managing the Care of People with Long-term Conditions: Second report of session 2014–2015,* p. 3, www.parliament.uk/business/committees/committees-a-z/commons-select/health-committee/inquiries/parliament-2010/long-term-conditions/

76 O'Carroll, R.E., *et al.*, 'Improving medication adherence in stroke survivors: Mediators and moderators of treatment effects', *Health Psychology*, 2014, 33: 1241–1250.

77 www.theheartmanual.com/Programmes/Pages/default.aspx

78 Johnston, Marie, *et al.*, 'Impact on patients and partners of inpatient and extended cardiac counselling and rehabilitation: A controlled trial', *Psychosomatic Medicine*, 1999, 61(2): 225–233.

79 www.nesta.org.uk/centre-social-action-innovation-fund-long-term-health-conditions

80 Simmons, David, *et al.*, 'Impact of community based peer support in Type 2 diabetes: A cluster randomised controlled trial of individual and/or group approaches', *PLoS One*, 2015, http://journals.plos.org/plosone/article?id=10.1371/journal.pone.0120277

81 See www.england.nhs.uk/ourwork/qual-clin-lead/diabetes-prevention/

82 Peers for Progress, *Global Evidence for Peer Support: Humanizing healthcare*, www.ipfcc.org/bestpractices/global-evidence-for-peer-support.pdf

83 www.royalfree.nhs.uk/news-media/news/google-deepmind-qa/

84 Yardley, Lucy, *et al.*, 'Current issues and future directions for digital intervention research', *American Journal of Preventive Medicine*, 2016, Nov, 51(5): 814–815.

85 Kippax, Susan, 'Effective HIV prevention: The indispensable role of social science', *Journal of the International AIDS Society*, 2012, 15(2): e17357, www.ncbi.nlm.nih.gov/pmc/articles/PMC3499803/; Fan, Liu, *et al.*, 'Interactivity, engagement, and technology dependence: Understanding users' technology utilisation behaviour', *Behaviour & Information Technology*, 2016, www.tandfonline.com/doi/full/10.1080/0144929X.2016.1199051

86 Yardley, Lucy, *et al.*, 'Understanding and promoting engagement with digital behavior change interventions', *American Journal of Preventive Medicine*, 2016, Nov, 51(5): 833–842; Perksi, Olga, *et al.*, 'Conceptualising engagement with digital behaviour change interventions: A systematic review using principles from critical interpretive synthesis', *Translational Behavioral Medicine*, 2016, http://link.springer.com/article/10.1007/s13142-016-0453-1

87 For instance, Appleby, John, 'How does NHS spending compare with health spending internationally?', The King's Fund, 2016, www.kingsfund.org.uk/blog/2016/01/how-does-nhs-spending-compare-health-spending-internationally; OECD, 'Hospital beds (indicator)', 2016, https://data.oecd.org/healtheqt/hospital-beds.htm; Kelly, Elaine, and French, Eric, 'The distribution of healthcare spending: an international comparison', IFS, 2016, www.ifs.org.uk/publications/8737

88 See, for instance, The UK Medical Careers Research Group (UKMCRG), University of Oxford, www.uhce.ox.ac.uk/ukmcrg/

89 Gawande, Awul, *The Checklist Manifesto: How to get things right*, Metropolitan Books, 2009.

90 Ibid.; 'The Checklist: If something so simple can transform intensive care, what else can it do?', *The New Yorker*, 2007, www.newyorker.com/magazine/2007/12/10/the-checklist

91 Dixon-Woods, Mary, *et al.*, 'Explaining Michigan: Developing an ex post theory of a quality improvement program', *Millbank Q*, 2011, 89(2), www.ncbi.nlm.nih.

gov/pubmed/21676020; National Academy of Sciences, 'The Hospital Checklist: How social science insights improve healthcare outcomes', 2016, www.nap.edu/read/23510/#slide1

92 Anthes, Emily, 'Hospital checklists are meant to save lives – so why do they often fail?', *Nature*, 2015, 523(7562), www.nature.com/news/hospital-checklists-are-meant-to-save-lives-so-why-do-they-often-fail-1.18057; Fixsen, Dean, *et al.*, *Implementation Research: A synthesis of the literature*, 2005, http://nirn.fpg.unc.edu/sites/nirn.fpg.unc.edu/files/resources/NIRN-MonographFull-01-2005.pdf; Ghate, Deborah, 'From programs to systems: Deploying implementation science and practice for sustained real world effectiveness in services for children and families', *Journal of Clinical Child & Adolescent Psychology*, 2015: 1537–4424, www.tandfonline.com/doi/pdf/10.1080/15374416.2015.1077449

93 Nilson, Per, 'Making sense of implementation: Theories, models and frameworks', *Implementation Science*, 2015, 10(53), https://implementationscience.biomedcentral.com/articles/10.1186/s13012-015-0242-0

94 Stone, Sheldon, *et al.*, 'Evaluation of the national Cleanyourhands Campaign to reduce *Staphylococcus Aureus* Bacteraemia and *Clostridium Difficile* infection in hospitals in England & Wales through improved hand hygiene: A four year prospective ecological interrupted time-series study', *BMJ*, 2012, 344: e3005, www.bmj.com/content/344/bmj.e3005

95 Fuller, Christopher, *et al.*, 'The Feedback Intervention Trial (FIT) – Improving hand-hygiene compliance in UK healthcare workers: A stepped wedge cluster randomized controlled trial', *PLoS One*, 2012, 7(10): e41617, http://journals.plos.org/plosone/article?id=10.1371/journal.pone.0041617

96 www.prescribinganalytics.com/

97 Davenport, Francesca, 'New tool to improve antibiotic prescribing in doctor surgeries', Imperial College London, 2016, www3.imperial.ac.uk/newsandeventspggrp/imperialcollege/newssummary/news_22-11-2016-12-16-56

98 Hallsworth, Michael, *et al.*, 'Provision of social norm feedback to high prescribers of antibiotics in general practice: A pragmatic national randomised controlled trial', *The Lancet*, 2016, 387: 1743–1752, www.thelancet.com/pdfs/journals/lancet/PIIS0140-6736(16)00215-4.pdf

99 Dreischulte, Tobias, *et al.*, 'Safer prescribing – A trial of education, informatics, and financial incentives', *The New England Journal of Medicine*, 2016, 374: 1053–1064, www.nejm.org/doi/full/10.1056/NEJMsa1508955?af=R&rss=currentIssue&#t=article

100 Clarkson, Jan E., *et al.*, 'Changing clinicians' behavior: A randomized controlled trial of fees and education', *Journal of Dental Research*, 2008, 87(7): 640–644.

101 Pittet, Didier, 'Improving adherence to hand hygiene practice: A multidisciplinary approach', *Emerging Infectious Diseases*, 2001, 7(2), www.nc.cdc.gov/eid/article/7/2/70-0234_article; Sproat, Lisa, *et al.*, 'A multicentre survey of hand hygiene practice in intensive care units', *Journal of Hospital Infection*, 1994, 26(2): 137–148, www.sciencedirect.com/science/article/pii/0195670194900574

102 Michie, Susan, 'Improving health by changing behaviour: Health professionals, the public and patients', 2013, https://medicine.dundee.ac.uk/sites/medicine.dundee.ac.uk/files/Professor%20Susan%20Michie.pdf

103 Stone, Sheldon, et al., 'Evaluation of the national Cleanyourhands Campaign to reduce *Staphylococcus Aureus* bacteraemia and *Clostridium Difficile* infection in hospitals in England and Wales by improved hand hygiene: A four year, prospective, ecological, interrupted time series study', *BMJ*, 2012, 344: e3005, www.bmj.com/content/344/bmj.e3005

104 Fuller, Christopher, et al., 'The Feedback Intervention Trial (FIT) – Improving hand hygeine compliance in UK healthcare workers: A stepped wedge cluster randomised controlled trial', *PLoS One*, 2012, 7(10): e41617, http://journals.plos.org/plosone/article?id=10.1371/journal.pone.0041617

105 Health Foundation, 'Environmental engineering to increase hand hygiene compliance', 2016, www.health.org.uk/programmes/behavioural-insights-research-programme/projects/environmental-engineering-increase-hand

106 Morris, Stephen, 'Impact of centralising acute stroke services in English metropolitan areas on mortality and length of hospital stay: Difference-in-differences analysis', *BMJ*, 2014, 349: g4757

107 Eurostat, 'Practising physicians, 2008 and 2013 (per 100,000 inhabitants)', 2015, http://ec.europa.eu/eurostat/statistics-explained/index.php/File:Practising_physicians,_2008_and_2013_(%C2%B9)_(per_100_000_inhabitants)_Health2015B.png

108 Imison, Candace, et al., 'Reshaping the workforce to deliver the care patients need', *Nuffield Trust*, 2016, www.nuffieldtrust.org.uk/publications/reshaping-the-workforce

109 Royal College of General Practitioners, 'The 2022 GP: A vision for General Practice in the future NHS', 2013, www.rcgp.org.uk/policy/rcgp-policy-areas/general-practice-2022.aspx

110 NHS England, 'General Practice forward view: Workforce plans', 2016, www.england.nhs.uk/commissioning/primary-care-comm/gp-action-plan/

111 National Audit Office, *The Management of Adult Diabetes Services in the NHS: Progress review*, 2015, www.nao.org.uk/wp-content/uploads/2015/10/The-management-of-adult-diabetes-services-in-the-NHS-progress-review.pdf

112 See www.haverstockhealth.com/services/integrated-practice-unit/

113 Morris, Stephen, 'Impact of centralising acute stroke services in English metropolitan areas on mortality and length of hospital stay: Difference-in-differences analysis', *BMJ*, 2014, 349: g4757, www.bmj.com/content/349/bmj.g4757

114 www.centrallondonccg.nhs.uk/media/24178/CLCCG-Cavendish-Skype-pilot-interim-report.pdf

115 Academy of Medical Sciences, *Health of the Public in 2040*, 2016, Annex III, pp. 111–112, www.acmedsci.ac.uk/policy/policy-projects/health-of-the-public-in-2040/

116 https://improvement.nhs.uk/resources/improvement-directory/

117 www.england.nhs.uk/ourwork/innovation/nia/

118   See, for example, NHS England, 'Planning, assuring and delivering service change for patients', 2015, www.england.nhs.uk/wp-content/uploads/2015/10/plan-ass-deliv-serv-chge.pdf

119   https://implementationscience.biomedcentral.com

120   www.povertyactionlab.org/

121   Examples include the National Implementation Science Network, in the US, http://implementation.fpg.unc.edu/sites/implementation.fpg.unc.edu/files/NIRN-Implementation DriversAssessingBestPractices.pdf; and the Global Implementation Initiative, https://globalimplementation.org/resources/

122   NHS England, 'New care models – vanguard sites', 2015, www.england.nhs.uk/ourwork/futurenhs/new-care-models/; House of Lords Science and Technology Committee, *Behaviour Change: Second report of session 2010–12,* www.parliament.uk/business/committees/committees-a-z/lords-select/science-and-technology-committee/inquiries/behaviour/

123   Ivers, Noah M., *et al.*, 'Audit and feedback: Effects on professional practice and health-care outcomes', *The Cochrane Database of Systematic Reviews,* 2012, 6: Cd000259, http://onlinelibrary.wiley.com/doi/10.1002/14651858.CD000259.pub3/abstract

124   Ivers, Noah M., *et al.*, 'Growing literature, stagnant science? Systematic review, meta-regression and cumulative analysis of audit and feedback interventions in healthcare', *Journal of General Internal Medicine,* 2014, 29(11): 1534–1541, www.ncbi.nlm.nih.gov/pmc/articles/PMC4238192/

125   Ivers, Noah M., *et al.*, 'No more "business as usual" with audit and feedback inter-ventions: Towards an agenda for a reinvigorated intervention', *Implementation Science (IS),* 2014, 9: 14, https://implementationscience.biomedcentral.com/articles/10.1186/1748-5908-9-14

126   Ivers, Noah M., and Grimshaw, Jeremy M., 'Reducing research waste with implementa-tion laboratories', *The Lancet,* 2016, 388(10044): 547–548.

127   Ham, Chris, and Aderwick, Hugh, *Place-based Systems of Care: A way forward for the NHS in England,* The King's Fund, 2015, www.kingsfund.org.uk/sites/files/kf/field/field_publication_file/Place-based-systems-of-care-Kings-Fund-Nov-2015_0.pdf; Alderwick, Hugh, Ham, Chris, and Buck, David, 'Population health systems: Going beyond integrated care', The King's Fund, 2015, www.kingsfund.org.uk/sites/files/kf/field/field_publication_file/population-health-systems-kingsfund-feb15.pdf

128   NHS Improving Quality, *Population Level Commissioning for the Future,* 2014, http://webarchive.nationalarchives.gov.uk/20160805125127/www.nhsiq.nhs.uk/media/2514788/population_level_commissioning_for_the_future.pdf; NHS England, *'How to' Guide: The BCF technical toolkit,* 2014, www.england.nhs.uk/wp-content/uploads/2014/09/1-seg-strat.pdf

129   Health Foundation, 'Applying hindsight to insight: Learning so far from our research programme on health informatics', 2016, www.health.org.uk/blog/applying-hindsight-insight-learning-so-far-our-research-programme-health-informatics

130 Academy of Medical Sciences, *Health of the Public in 2040*, 2016, www.acmedsci. ac.uk/policy/policy-projects/health-of-the-public-in-2040/

131 See http://tdi.dartmouth.edu/

132 Alderwick, Hugh, *et al.*, *Better Value in the NHS: The role of changes in clinical practice*, The King's Fund, 2015, p. 9, www.kingsfund.org.uk/sites/files/kf/field/field_publication_file/ better-value-nhs-Kings-Fund-July%202015.pdf

133 See the UK Statistics Authority, 'Health and care statistics in England – The Statistics Authority's direction of travel', 2016, www.statisticsauthority.gov.uk/wp-content/ uploads/2016/03/Health-statistics-direction-of-travel.pdf

134 Wachter, Robert, *Making IT Work: Harnessing the power of health information technology to improve care in England,* 2016, www.gov.uk/government/uploads/system/uploads/ attachment_data/file/550866/Wachter_Review_Accessible.pdf

135 Ibid., p. 16.

136 French, Eric, and Kelly, Elaine, *The Distribution of Healthcare Spending: An international comparison*, Institute for Fiscal Studies, 2016, www.ifs.org.uk/publications/8737; French, Eric, and Kelly, Elaine, 'Medical spending around the developed world', *Fiscal Studies*, 2016, 37: 327–344, doi:10.1111/j.1475-5890.2016.12127

137 These are based on the definitions in the Information Commissioner's Office Anonymisation Code of Practice: https://ico.org.uk/for-organisations/guide-to-data-protection/anonymisation/

138 Caldicott, Fiona, *National Data Guardian for Health Care Review of Data Security, Consent and Opt-Outs*, 2016, www.gov.uk/government/uploads/system/uploads/ attachment_data/file/535024/data-security-review.PDF

139 National Audit Office, *Stocktake of Access to General Practice in England,* 2015, www. nao.org.uk/wp-content/uploads/2015/11/Stocktake-of-access-to-general-practice-in-England.pdf

140 Productivity Commission, *Data Availability and Use*, Draft Report, 2016, www.pc.gov. au/inquiries/current/data-access/draft/data-access-draft.pdf; Desai, Tanvi, *et al.*, *Five Safes: Designing data access for research*, Economics Working Paper Series, University of the West of England, 2016, www1.uwe.ac.uk/bl/research/bristoleconomicanalysis/ economicsworkingpapers/economicspapers2016.aspx; and Moody, Victoria, 'Access to sensitive data for research: "The 5 Safes"', UK Data Services, 2015, http://blog. ukdataservice.ac.uk/access-to-sensitive-data-for-research-the-5-safes/

141 Ipsos MORI, *Dialogue on Data: Exploring the public's views on using administrative data for research purposes*, 2014, www.ipsos-mori.com/Assets/Docs/Publications/sri-dialogue-on-data-2014.pdf;

142 Ipsos MORI, *The One-Way Mirror: Public attitudes to commercial access to health data*, 2016, www.ipsos-mori.com/Assets/Docs/Publications/sri-wellcome-trust-commercial-access-to-health-data.pdf

143 www.england.nhs.uk/ourwork/tsd/care-data/

144 Wellcome Trust, 'Independent patient data taskforce announced', 2016, https://wellcome.ac.uk/news/independent-patient-data-taskforce-announced%20

145 www.ukcrc.org/research-coordination/joint-funding-initiatives/public-health-research/

146 www.nihr.ac.uk/about-us/how-we-are-managed/our-structure/research/health-protection-research-units.htm

147 www.bhru.iph.cam.ac.uk/

148 www.mrc.ac.uk/research/initiatives/national-prevention-research-initiative-npri/

149 www.ucl.ac.uk/behaviour-change

150 www.health.org.uk/creating-new-improvement-research-institute-0

151 Department of Health, *Innovation, Health and Wealth*, 2011, http://webarchive.nationalarchives.gov.uk/20130107105354/http:/www.dh.gov.uk/prod_consum_dh/groups/dh_digitalassets/documents/digitalasset/dh_134597.pdf

152 See, for example, www.ahsnnetwork.com/new-atlas-solutions-healthcare-aims-help-speed-adoption-innovation/

153 See recommendations in Academy of Medical Sciences, *Improving the Health of the Public by 2040,* 2016.

154 Norman Freshney Consulting, 'UK research landscape for population health research and public health practice: Report for the Academy of Medical Sciences', 2016, www.acmedsci.ac.uk/snip/uploads/57f23c7da653c.pdf

155 Foy, Robbie, Eccles, Martin, and Grimshaw, Jeremy, 'Why does primary care need more implementation research?', *Family Practice*, 2001,18: 353–355, https://fampra.oxfordjournals.org/content/18/4/353.full

156 Prasad, V., and Ioannidis, J.P.A., 'Evidence-based de-implementation for contradicted, unproven, and aspiring healthcare practices', *Implementation Science*, 2014, 9: 1.

157 Ivers, Noah M., *et al.*, 'Audit and feedback: Effects on professional practice and healthcare outcomes', *The Cochrane Database of Systematic Reviews*, 2012, 6: Cd000259, http://onlinelibrary.wiley.com/doi/10.1002/14651858.CD000259.pub3/abstract

158 Ivers, Noah M., *et al.*, 'No more "business as usual" with audit and feedback interventions: Towards an agenda for a reinvigorated intervention', *Implementation Science (IS)*, 2014, 9: 14, https://implementationscience.biomedcentral.com/articles/10.1186/1748-5908-9-14

159 www.hee.nhs.uk/

160 Health Education England, 'Making every contact count', https://hee.nhs.uk/our-work/hospitals-primary-community-care/prevention-public-health-wellbeing/making-every-contact-count; NHS Education for Scotland, 'What is the Health Promoting Health Service (HPHS?)', www.knowledge.scot.nhs.uk/home/portals-and-topics/health-improvement/hphs.aspx; Public Health Wales, 'Making every contact count', www.knowledge.scot.nhs.uk/home/portals-and-topics/health-improvement/hphs.aspx

161 General Medical Council, *Tomorrow's Doctors: Recommendations on undergraduate medical education*, GMC, London, 2003.

162 Peters, Sarah, and Livia, Andrea, 'Relevant behavioural and social science for medical undergraduates: A comparison of specialist and non-specialist educators', *Medical Education*, 2006, 40(10): 1020–1026, http://onlinelibrary.wiley.com/doi/10.1111/j.1365-2929.2006.02562.x/abstract

163 Alder, Beth, *et al.*, *Psychology and Sociology Applied to Medicine*, Elsevier Health Sciences, 2011; Goodman, Benny, *Psychology and Sociology in Nursing*, Learning Matters, 2015.

164 Dixon, Diane, and Johnston, Marie, *Health Behaviour Change Competency Framework: Competences to deliver interventions to change lifestyle behaviours that affect health*, NHS Health Scotland, 2010, www.healthscotland.com/uploads/documents/4877-Health_behaviour_change_competency_framework.pdf

165 https://elearning.healthscotland.com/course/index.php?categoryid=108

166 Academy of Medical Sciences, 'Health of the Public in 2040', 2016, p. 8, www.acmedsci.ac.uk/policy/policy-projects/health-of-the-public-in-2040/

167 House of Commons, Health and Social Care (National Data Guardian) Bill 2016–17, www.publications.parliament.uk/pa/bills/cbill/2016-2017/0084/cbill_2016-20170084_en_2.htm#pb1-l1g; House of Commons, Digital Economy Bill (HC Bill 45), chapter 5, www.publications.parliament.uk/pa/bills/cbill/2016-2017/0045/cbill_2016-20170045_en_1.htm

168 Wellcome Trust, 'Sharing research data to improve public health: Full joint statement by funders of health research', https://wellcome.ac.uk/what-we-do/our-work/sharing-research-data-improve-public-health-full-joint-statement-funders-health

169 See recommendation 2: Academy of Medical Sciences, *Health of the Public in 2040*, 2016, www.acmedsci.ac.uk/policy/policy-projects/health-of-the-public-in-2040/